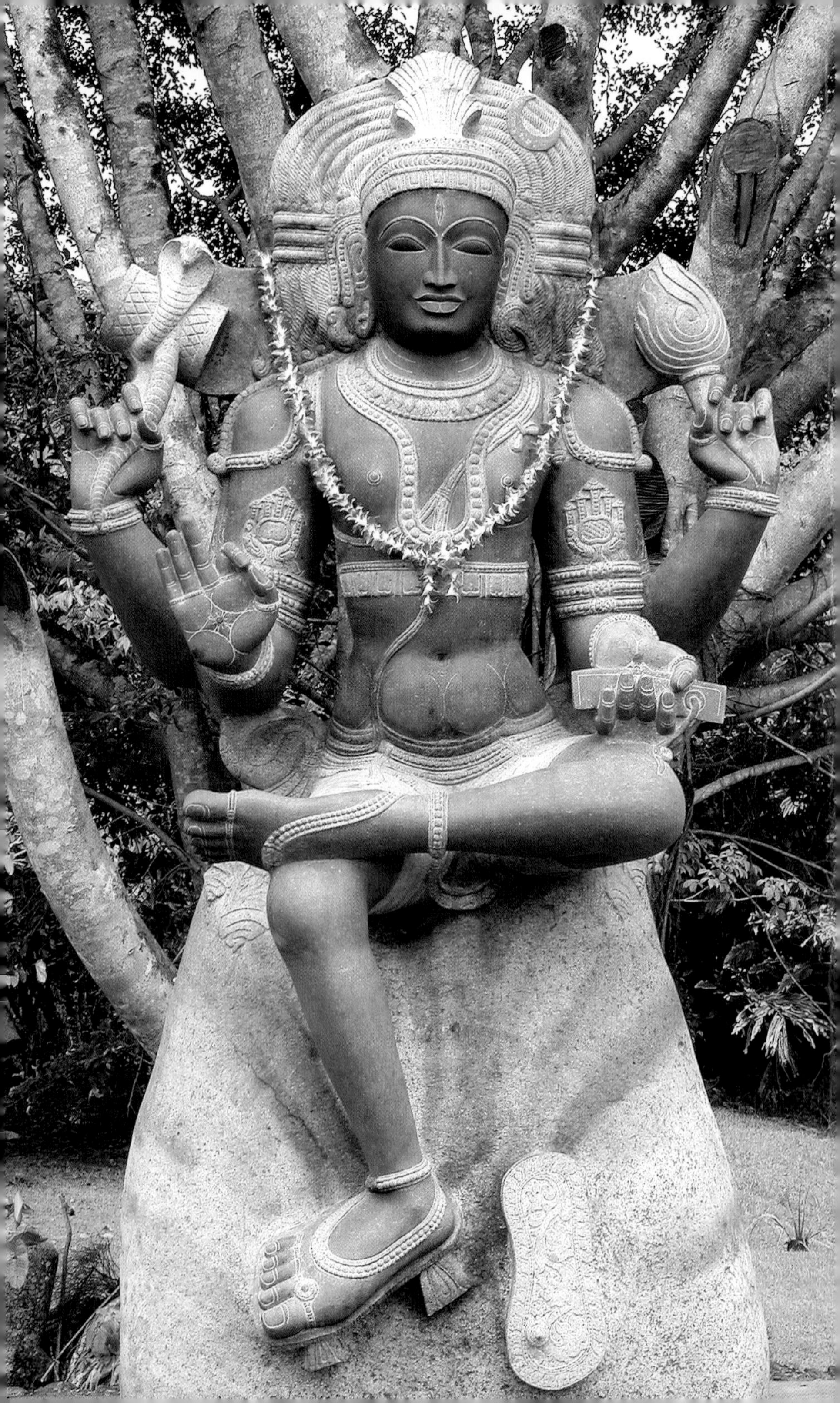

Yoga's Forgotten Foundation

विस्मृतम् योगस्य मूलम्

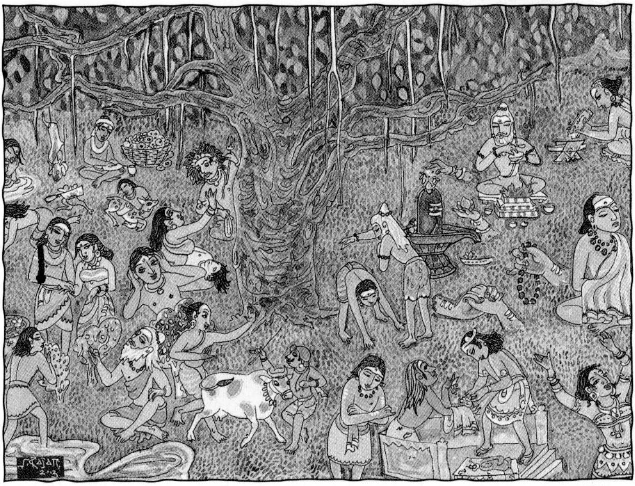

First Edition

Published by
Himalayan Academy
USA • India

PRINTED IN MALAYSIA BY SAMPOORNA PRINTERS SDN BHD
BY ARRANGEMENT WITH UMA PUBLICATIONS

Library of Congress Control Number 2003110985
ISBN 0-945497-91-1

Art Descriptions

Chapter Art: The art opening each chapter is the work of A. Manivelu.

Cover Art: Artist S. Rajam depicts Lord Śiva embracing the restraints and observances with ten pairs of seekers, one yama *and one* niyama *as described in the text.*

Dakshiṇāmūrti: Opposite the half-title page is a photo of the twelve-foot-tall black granite statue of Lord Śiva as the silent sage, teacher of teachers. The statue is situated at Kauai's Hindu Monastery at the north perimeter of Iraivan Temple.

Half-title page: S. Rajam paints each of the twenty yamas *and* niyamas *being practiced under a giant forest tree.*

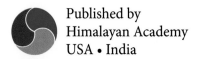

Yoga's Forgotten Foundation

Twenty Timeless Keys To Your Divine Destiny

विस्मृतम् योगस्य मूलम्

ध्यानार्थं सौभाग्यदाः विंशति-कालातित-सूक्तयः

Satguru Sivaya Subramuniyaswami

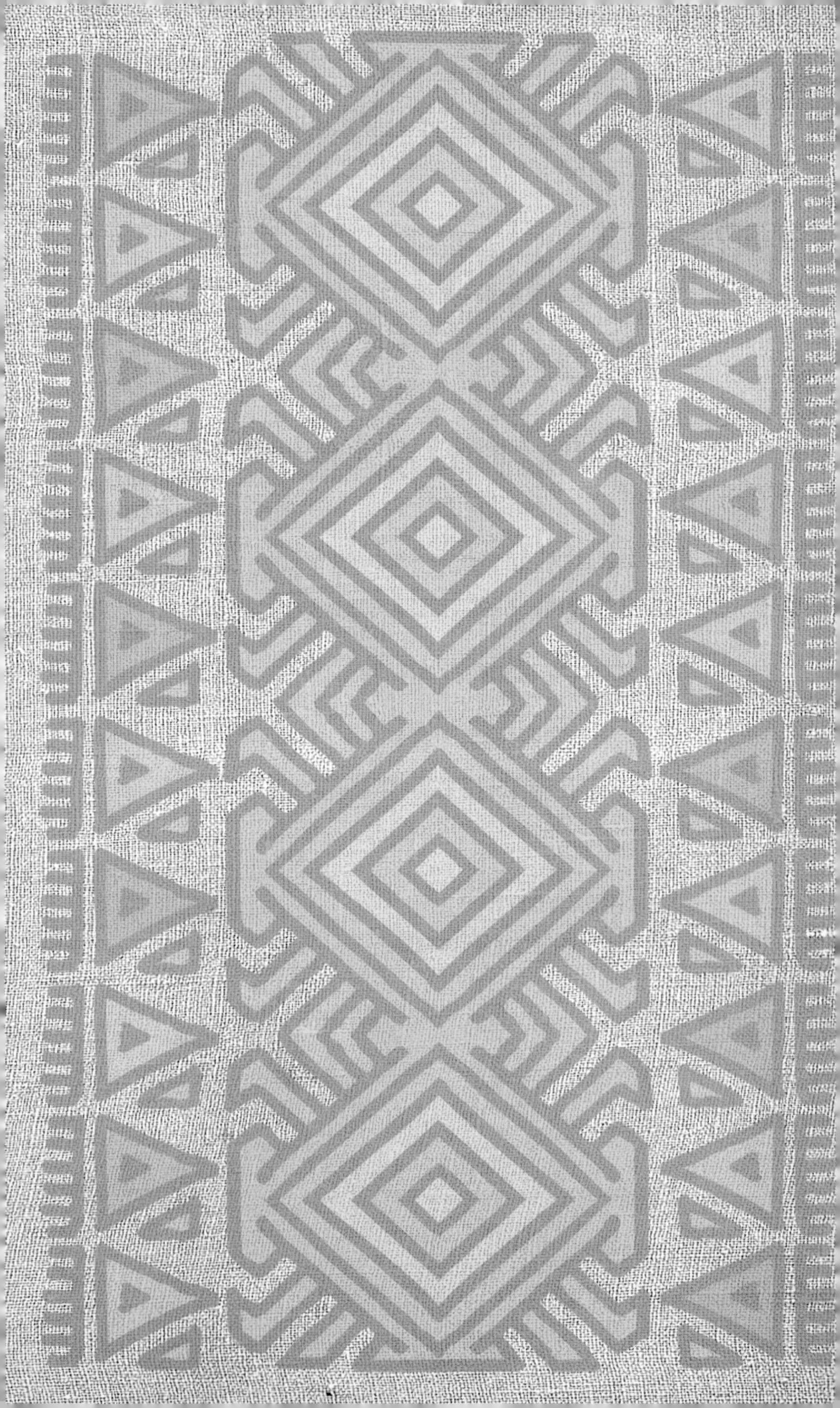

Contents

Vishayasūchi विषयसूची

Foreword

Upakramaḥ उपक्रमः

GURUDEVA TRAVELED BY AIR OFTEN, AND FROM TIME TO TIME COMMENTED ON HOW PROFESSIONALLY THE FLIGHT CREW HAD CONDUCTED THEMSELVES. HE WOULD ASK, "HOW often do you see a professional team of people misbehave on the job? You're on a flight from San Francisco to Singapore. Do the stewardesses bicker in the aisle? Of course not. People at this level of business have control of their minds and emotions. If they didn't, they would soon be replaced. When they are on the job, at least, they follow a code of conduct spelled out in detail by the corporation." He would go on to say that it's not unlike the moral code of any religion, outlining sound ethics for respect and harmony among humans. Those seeking to be successful in life strive to fulfill a moral code whether "on the job" or off. Does Hinduism and its scriptures on *yoga* have such a code? Yes: twenty ethical guidelines called *yamas* and *niyamas,* "restraints and observances."

These "do's" and "don'ts" are a common-sense code recorded in the *Upanishads,* the final section of the 6,000- to 8,000-year-old *Vedas,* mankind's oldest body of scripture, and in other holy texts expounding the path of *yoga.* The *yamas* and *niyamas* have been preserved through the centuries as the foundation, the first and second stages, of the eight-staged practice of *yoga.* Yet, they are fundamental to all beings, expected aims of everyone in society, and assumed to be fully intact for anyone seeking life's highest aim in the pursuit called *yoga.* Sage Patanjali (ca 200 BCE), *raja yoga's* foremost propounder, told us, "These *yamas* are not limited by class, country, time (past, present or future) or situation. Hence they are called the universal great vows." *Yogic* scholar

Swami Brahmananda Saraswati revealed the inner science of *yama* and *niyama.* They are the means, he said, to control the *vitarkas,* the cruel mental waves or thoughts, that when acted upon result in injury to others, untruthfulness, hoarding, discontent, indolence or selfishness. He stated, "For each *vitarka* you have, you can create its opposite through *yama* and *niyama,* and make your life successful."

Today's popular concept of *yoga* equates it with *haṭha yoga* and the practice of the *haṭha yoga āsanas,* or postures. Many who practice yoga do so solely for health benefits. However, others pursue it in hopes of reaping the spiritual benefits it offers. It is to these spiritual seekers who have higher consciousness as the goal of their *yoga* that this book is directed.

Yoga is also known as *ashṭāṅga yoga* because it consists of eight stages: *yama,* restraint; *niyama,* observance; *āsana,* seat or posture; *prāṇāyāma,* mastering life force; *pratyāhāra,* withdrawal; *dharaṇā,* concentration; *dhyāna,* meditation; and *samādhi,* God Realization. These two vital stages—*yama,* the restraints; and *niyama,* the observances—traditionally precede *āsana,* but they are omitted in most *yoga* classes today. We can liken these eight limbs to a tall building. The *yamas* are the first part of the foundation, like the cement, and the *niyamas* are the second part, like the steel. Together they provide the support a skyscraper needs to stand. *Āsana, prāṇāyāma* and *pratyāhāra* are like the lower floors, *dhāraṇa, dhyāna,* the middle ones, and *samādhi* is the top floor.

I remember years ago watching the Transamerica Building in San Francisco being erected. First the construction crew dug down quite a depth with huge equipment. Then massive steel pilings were driven, inches at a time, hundreds of feet into the earth. Then thousands of yards of concrete were poured. The long lineup of cement trucks created a traffic jam in the well-trafficked business district. From the concrete, the steel rose upward as a framework for the rest of the structure. This massive foundation was needed to keep this famous modern pyramid from toppling in an earthquake.

In spiritual life, without a foundation of good character and discipline, success in *yoga* will not be lasting. Sooner or later, the earthquakes in our personal life, the times of great stress and difficulty, will bring outbursts of anger or periods of discouragement, causing our higher consciousness to fall back to Earth. To quote from Gurudeva: "It is true that bliss comes from meditation, and it is true that higher consciousness is the heritage of all mankind. However, the ten restraints and their corresponding practices are necessary to maintain bliss consciousness." We are a soul, a divine being, and it is important to reflect on that Divinity. However, we are living in a physical body, and, therefore, in addition to the soul, we also have an instinctive and intellectual nature. Gurudeva describes this as the three phases of the mind: instinctive, intellectual and superconscious.

Making progress on the spiritual path requires learning to control the instinctive mind. This is where the *yamas* come into play. They give us a list of tendencies we need to control. The classical depiction of restraint is the charioteer pulling back on the reins of a team of horses to keep them under control. The practice of the niyamas develops a more cultured nature that takes joy in scriptural study, devotional practices and helping others. It focuses on expressing our soul nature in our outer actions. Together the yamas and niyamas provide the foundation to support our yoga practice so that attainments in higher consciousness can be sustained.

How Gurudeva Created this Book

Yoga's Forgotten Foundation was dictated by Satguru Sivaya Subramuniyaswami during twenty-five afternoon editing sessions with two of his *āchāryas* at Kauai's Beachboy Hotel between February 14 and March 26, 1990. Gurudeva was determined to capture the essence of these ancient guidelines and bring them forward to the world in answer to the fallacy that "Hinduism has no code of ethics." For many decades, he had known only of the five *yamas* and *niyamas* that are presented by Sage Patanjali in his *Yoga Sūtras* and brushed over in nearly all yoga texts as the first and second stages of *ashṭāṅga yoga.* But those ten guidelines were not complete enough to encompass the broad scope of human conduct. In the late sixties, in fact, Gurudeva presented his own unique 36-point code of virtuous, contemplative living, which included planting trees, perfecting an art or craft and leaving beauty where you pass (see *Living with Śiva* chapter 14, "Life the Great Experience"). So, finding that there was indeed an ancient and much more comprehensive set of twenty *yamas* and *niyamas* was like unearthing gold. His swamis discovered these in Rishi Tirumular's *Tirumantiram*, a 2,200-year-old yogic scripture written in ancient Tamil, which Gurudeva commissioned Dr. B. Natarajan to translate into English in 1978. Now they had only to be elucidated and brought into the Hindu mainstream through cogent commentary.

From the outset, Gurudeva envisioned his dissertations being compiled into a book—the very book you now hold in your hands. Sitting with his monastic editing team from 4 to 7pm every day for five weeks, Gurudeva spoke out from the "inner sky" on each virtue and religious practice, responding to specific questions from the two *āchāryas* to draw forth his wisdom. Gurudeva used to say, "I have good writers upstairs." The answers were typed into the very first laptop computer we ever owned, a Sony TypeCorder, which recorded the text on micro-cassette tapes, which were downloaded to desktop Macintoshes at the monastery the next day. At that time, there were lots of other projects in process for the Ganapati Kulam (the monastery group that produces publications), most importantly *Dancing with Śiva*, so all those hours of dictation were neatly set aside for some future date when they could be compiled, cleaned up (it was horribly difficult to type on that stiff Sony keyboard) and brought back to the table for editing suggestions and for further input from Gurudeva. As unlikely as it would have seemed then, those precious manuscripts would lie untouched for a full ten years, until the turn of the millennium, when Gurudeva turned his attention to *Living with Śiva,* the third massive tome in his Master Course trilogy. In fact, Gurudeva considered these *yamas* and *niyamas* the heart and core of that thousand-page masterpiece on Hinduism's contemporary culture. He worked on *Living with Śiva* at his editing sessions every day for almost two years, beginning in 1999, driven inwardly to complete it.

It was only after Gurudeva's passing into the Śivaloka in 2001 that the idea reemerged of a separate small book presenting this ancient and now fully illuminated "code of conduct." I was inspired to extract and repurpose it to reach a broader audience as a handbook for spiritual life. Like Gurudeva, I was concerned that so many seekers are unaware of these guidelines for good character and self-discipline and therefore are not properly prepared for the practice of *yoga,* or even to live a wholesome, spiritual life.

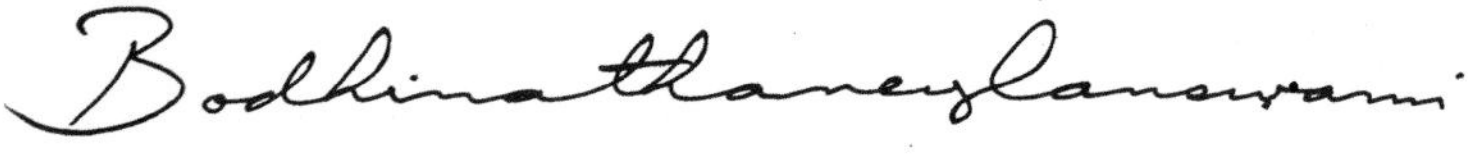

Satguru Bodhinatha Veylanswami
163rd Jagadāchārya of the Nandinātha
Sampradāya's Kailāsa Paramparā
Guru Mahāsannidhānam
Kauai Aadheenam, Hawaii

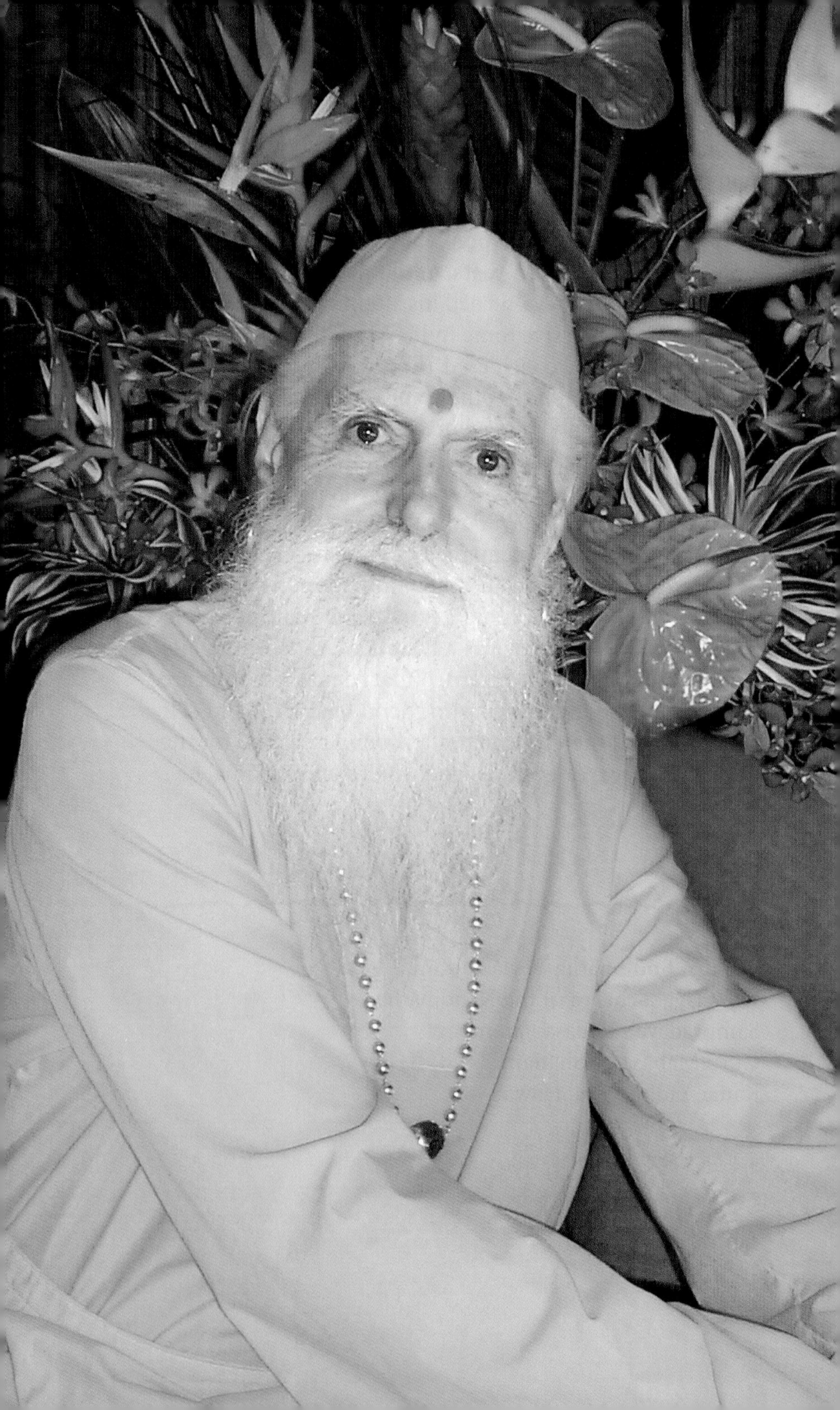

Introduction

Bhūmikā भूमिका

RELIGION TEACHES US HOW TO BECOME BETTER PEOPLE, HOW TO LIVE AS SPIRITUAL BEINGS ON THIS EARTH. THIS HAPPENS THROUGH LIVING VIRTUOUSLY, FOLLOWING the natural and essential guidelines of *dharma.* For Hindus, these guidelines are recorded in the *yamas* and *niyamas,* ancient scriptural injunctions for all aspects of human thought, attitude and behavior. In Indian spiritual life, these Vedic restraints and observances are built into the character of children from a very early age. For adults who have been subjected to opposite behavioral patterns, these guidelines may seem to be like commandments. However, even they can, with great dedication and effort, remold their character and create the foundation necessary for a sustained spiritual life. Through following the *yamas* and *niyamas,* we cultivate our refined, spiritual being while keeping the instinctive nature in check. We lift ourself into the consciousness of the higher *chakras*—of love, compassion, intelligence and bliss—and naturally invoke the blessings of the divine *devas* and Mahādevas.

Yama means "reining in" or "control." The *yamas* include such injunctions as noninjury *(ahiṁsā),* nonstealing *(asteya)* and moderation in eating *(mitāhāra),* which harness the base, instinctive nature. *Niyama,* literally "unleashing," indicates the expression of refined, soul qualities through such disciplines as charity *(dāna),* contentment *(santosha)* and incantation *(japa).*

It is true that bliss comes from meditation, and it is true that higher consciousness is the heritage of all mankind. However, the ten restraints and their corresponding practices are necessary to maintain bliss consciousness, as well as all of the good feelings toward oneself and others attainable in any incarnation. These restraints and practices build character. Character is the foundation for spiritual unfoldment.

The fact is, the higher we go, the lower we can fall. The top *chakras* spin fast; the lowest one available to us spins even faster. The platform of character must be built within our lifestyle to maintain the total contentment needed to persevere on the path. These great *ṛishis* saw the frailty of human nature and gave these guidelines, or disciplines, to make it strong. They said, "Strive!" Let's strive to not hurt others, to be truthful and honor all the rest of the virtues they outlined.

The ten *yamas* are: 1) *ahiṁsā,* "noninjury," not harming others by thought, word or deed; 2) *satya,* "truthfulness," refraining from lying and betraying promises; 3) *asteya,* "nonstealing," neither stealing nor coveting nor entering into debt; 4) *brahmacharya,* "divine conduct," controlling lust by remaining celibate when single, leading to faithfulness in marriage; 5) *kshamā,* "patience," restraining intolerance with people and impatience with circumstances; 6) *dhṛiti,* "steadfastness," overcoming nonperseverance, fear, indecision, inconstancy and changeableness; 7) *dayā,* "compassion," conquering callous, cruel and insensitive feelings toward all beings; 8) *ārjava,* "honesty, straightforwardness," renouncing deception and wrongdoing; 9) *mitāhāra,* "moderate appetite," neither eating too much nor consuming meat, fish, fowl or eggs; 10) *śaucha,* "purity," avoiding impurity in body, mind and speech.

The *niyamas* are: 1) *hrī,* "remorse," being modest and showing shame for misdeeds; 2) *santosha,* "contentment," seeking joy and serenity in life; 3) *dāna,* "giving," tithing and giving generously without thought of reward; 4) *āstikya,* "faith," believing firmly in God, Gods, *guru* and the path to enlightenment; 5) Īśvarapūjana, "worship of the Lord," the cultivation of devotion through daily worship and meditation; 6) *siddhānta śravaṇa,* "scriptural listening," studying the teachings and listening to the wise of one's lineage; 7) *mati,* "cognition," developing a spiritual will and intellect with the *guru's* guidance; 8) *vrata,* "sacred vows," fulfilling religious vows, rules and observances faithfully; 9) *japa,* "recitation," chanting *mantras* daily; 10) *tapas,* "austerity," performing *sādhana,* penance, *tapas* and sacrifice.

In comparing the *yamas* to the *niyamas,* we find the restraint of noninjury, *ahiṁsā,* makes it possible to practice *hrī,* remorse. Truthfulness brings on the state of *santosha,* contentment. And the third *yama, asteya,* nonstealing, must be perfected before the third *niyama,* giving without any thought of reward, is even possible. Sexual purity brings faith in God, Gods and *guru. Kshamā,* patience, is the foundation for Īśvarapūjana, worship, as is *dhṛiti,* steadfastness, the foundation for *siddhānta śravana.* The *yama* of *dayā,* compassion, definitely brings *mati,* cognition. *Ārjava,* honesty—renouncing deception and all wrongdoing—is the foundation for *vrata,* taking sacred vows and faithfully fulfilling them. *Mitāhāra,* moderate appetite, is where *yoga* begins, and vegetarianism is essential before the practice of *japa,* recitation of holy *mantras,* can reap its true benefit in one's life. *Śaucha,* purity in body, mind and speech, is the foundation and the protection for all austerities.

The twenty restraints and observances are the first two of the eight limbs of *ashṭāṅga yoga,* constituting Hinduism's fundamental ethical code. Because it is brief, the entire code can be easily memorized and reviewed daily at the family meetings in each home. The *yamas* and *niyamas* are the essential foundation for all spiritual progress. They are cited in numerous scriptures, including the *Śāṇḍilya* and *Varāha Upanishads,* the *Haṭha Yoga Pradīpikā* by Gorakshanatha, the *Tirumantiram* of Rishi Tirumular and the *Yoga Sūtras* of Sage Patanjali. All of these ancient texts list ten *yamas* and ten *niyamas*, with the exception of Patanjali's classic work, which lists just five of each. Patanjali lists the *yamas* as: *ahiṁsā, satya, asteya, brahmacharya* and *aparigraha* (non-covetousness); and the *niyamas* as: *śaucha, santosha, tapas, svādhyāya* (self-reflection, scriptural study) and *Īśvarapraṇidhāna* (worship).

In the Hindu tradition, it is primarily the mother's job to build character within the children, and thereby to continually improve society. Mothers can study and teach these guidelines to uplift their children as well as themselves. Each discipline focuses on a different aspect of human nature, its strengths and weaknesses. Taken as a sum total, they encompass the whole of human experience and spirituality. You may do well in upholding some of these but not so well in others. That is to be expected. That defines the *sādhana*, therefore, to be perfected.

The *yamas* and *niyamas* and their function in our life can be likened to a chariot pulled by ten horses. The passenger inside the chariot is your soul. The chariot itself represents your physical, astral and mental bodies. The driver of the chariot is your external ego, your personal will. The wheels are your divine energies. The *niyamas,* or spiritual practices, represent the spirited horses, named Hrī, Santosha, Dāna, Āstikya, Īśvarapūjana, Siddhānta Śravaṇa, Mati, Vrata, Japa, and Tapas. The *yamas,* or restraints, are the reins, called Ahiṁsā, Satya, Asteya, Brahmacharya, Kshamā, Dhṛiti, Dayā, Ārjava, Mitāhāra and Śaucha. By holding tight to the reins, the charioteer, your will, guides the strong horses so they can run forward swiftly and gallantly as a dynamic unit. So, as we restrain the lower, instinctive qualities through upholding the *yamas,* the soul moves forward to its destination in the state of *santosha. Santosha*, peace, is the eternal satisfaction of the soul. At the deepest level, the soul is always in the state of *santosha.* But outwardly, the propensity of the soul is to be clouded by lack of restraint of the instinctive nature, lack of restraint of the intellectual nature, lack of restraint of the emotional nature, lack of restraint of the physical body itself. Therefore, hold tight the reins.

The *yamas,* or restraints, must be well understood and accomplished before the *niyamas* can be earnestly undertaken. While we are worried about truthfulness, nonstealing, patience, compassion and being honest, how can we practice the *niyamas*—contentment, charity, worship, recitation of *mantras?* The answer is, we can't. The *niyamas* follow the *yamas.* Once the *yamas* are safely tucked away, and our lifestyle, thinking style, speech style, emotional style reflect these ten restaints, then we can move on to the *niyamas.* Once you feel you have a minimal mastery of the *yamas,* then go on to the *niyamas,* the practices, in full vigor. The observances will strengthen the restraints, as the restraints will allow us to fulfill the observances.

You must realize that throughout this process you are a self-effulgent soul, perfect in every way, incomprehensibly beautiful, as a shining one, but that the lifestyles, thinking styles, etc., at this time in the Kali Yuga are incomprehensibly complex, often demoralizing, and depression can set in at a moment's notice. But always keep in mind your here-and-now perfection, already-done perfection. You don't have to do a thing about it other than learn how to live with it, and manifest it in your daily life. Deal with it. These restraints and observances can adjust the outside view to the beautiful self-effulgent, shining inner you.

It is important to realize that the *yamas,* restraints, are not out of the reach of the lowliest among us. No matter where we are in the scale of life, we all started from the beginning, at the bottom, didn't we? This is our philosophy. This is our religion. This is the evolution of the soul. We improve, life after life, and these guidelines, *yamas* and *niyamas,* restraints and practices, are gifts from our *ṛishis,* from God Śiva Himself through them, to allow us to judge ourself against these pillars of virtue as to how far we have progressed or strayed. In the early births, we are like children. We do not stray from anything. We run here and there and everywhere, disobey every rule, which when told of we cannot remember. We ignore any admonishment. As adolescents, we force our will on society, want to change it, because we don't like the hold it has on us. Wanting to express themselves in most creative ways, rebellious youths separate themselves from other people, children and the adults. They do make changes, but not always for the best. As an adult, we see both—the past and the impending future of old age—and, heads down, we are concerned with accumulating enough to see life through to its uncertain end. When the accumulations have become adequate, we will look back at the undisciplined children, the headstrong, unruly adolescents and the self-possessed, concentrated adults and try to motivate all three groups. In our great religion, the Sanātana Dharma, known today as Hinduism, twenty precepts, the *yamas* and *niyamas,* restraints and observances, are the guidelines we use to motivate these three groups. These are the guidelines they use to motivate themselves, for each group is mystically independent of the others; so it seems.

The Way of Yama-Niyama
The Being First,
The Meaning-Central of *Vedas* all,
The Light Divine,
The Fire within that Light,
He who shares Himself
Half-and-Half with His Śakti
And the Divine Justice thereof—
Them, he in *niyama's* path knows.

Ten Virtues of Yama
Purity, compassion, frugal food and patience
Forthrightness, truth and steadfastness—
These he ardently cherishes.
Killing, stealing and lusting he abhors.
Thus stands with virtues ten
The one who *niyama's* ways observes.

Ten Attributes of Niyama
Tapas, meditation, serenity, and holiness
Charity, vows in Śaiva Way and Siddhānta learning
Sacrifice, Śiva *pūjā* and thoughts pure—
With these ten, the one in
Niyama perfects his Ways.

Tirumantiram, 555-557

The Ten *Yamas,* Restraints for Proper Conduct from the *Vedas*

1. Noninjury, *ahiṁsā:* Not harming others by thought, word, or deed.
2. Truthfulness, *satya:* Refraining from lying and betraying promises.
3. Nonstealing, *asteya:* Neither stealing, nor coveting nor entering into debt.
4. Divine conduct, *brahmacharya:* Controlling lust by remaining celibate when single, leading to faithfulness in marriage.
5. Patience, *kshamā:* Restraining intolerance with people and impatience with circumstances.
6. Steadfastness, *dhṛiti:* Overcoming nonperseverance, fear, indecision and changeableness.
7. Compassion, *dayā:* Conquering callous, cruel and insensitive feelings toward all beings.
8. Honesty, straightforwardness, *ārjava:* Renouncing deception and wrongdoing.
9. Moderate appetite, *mitāhāra:* Neither eating too much nor consuming meat, fish, fowl or eggs.
10. Purity, *śaucha:* Avoiding impurity in body, mind and speech.

The Ten *Niyamas,* Observances For Spiritual Life from the *Vedas*

1. Remorse, *hrī:* Being modest and showing shame for misdeeds.
2. Contentment, *santosha:* Seeking joy and serenity in life.
3. Giving, *dāna:* Tithing and giving generously without thought of reward.
4. Faith, *āstikya:* Believing firmly in God, Gods, *guru* and the path to enlightenment.
5. Worship of the Lord, *Īśvarapūjana:* The cultivation of devotion through daily worship and meditation.
6. Scriptural listening, *siddhānta śravaṇa:* Studying the teachings and listening to the wise of one's lineage.
7. Cognition, *mati:* Developing a spiritual will and intellect with the guru's guidance.
8. Sacred vows, *vrata:* Fulfilling religious vows, rules and observances faithfully.
9. Recitation, *japa:* Chanting *mantras* daily.
10. Austerity, *tapas:* Performing *sādhana,* penance, *tapas* and sacrifice.

One man is beating a small boy, while an onlooker rushes forward to intervene and stop the injury.

Summary of the First Restraint

Practice noninjury, not harming others by thought, word or deed, even in your dreams. Live a kindly life, revering all beings as expressions of the One Divine energy. Let go of fear and insecurity, the sources of abuse. Knowing that harm caused to others unfailingly returns to oneself, live peacefully with God's creation. Never be a source of dread, pain or injury. Follow a vegetarian diet.

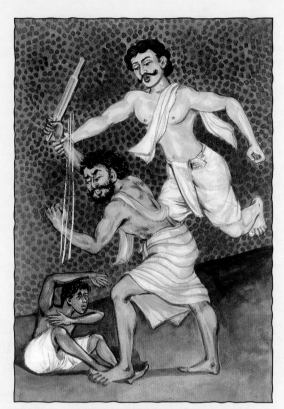

THE FIRST RESTRAINT

Noninjury

Ahiṁsā अहिंसा

THE FIRST *YAMA* IS *AHIṀSĀ*, NONINJURY. TO PRACTICE *AHIṀSĀ*, ONE HAS TO PRACTICE *SANTOSHA*, CONTENTMENT. THE *SĀDHANA* IS TO SEEK JOY AND SERENITY IN LIFE, REmaining content with what one has, knows, is doing and those with whom he associates. Bear your *karma* cheerfully. Live within your situation contentedly. *Hiṁsā,* or injury, and the desire to harm, comes from discontent.

The *ṛishis* who revealed the principles of *dharma* or divine law in Hindu scripture knew full well the potential for human suffering and the path which could avert it. To them a one spiritual power flowed in and through all things in this universe, animate and inanimate, conferring existence by its presence. To them life was a coherent process leading all souls without exception to enlightenment, and no violence could be carried to the higher reaches of that ascent. These *ṛishis* were mystics whose revelation disclosed a cosmos in which all beings exist in interlaced dependence. The whole is contained in the part, and the part in the whole. Based on this cognition, they taught a philosophy of nondifference of self and other, asserting that in the final analysis we are not separate from the world and its manifest forms, nor from the Divine which shines forth in all things, all beings, all peoples. From this understanding of oneness arose the philosophical basis for the practice of noninjury and Hinduism's ancient commitment to it.

We all know that Hindus, who are one-sixth of the human race today, believe in the existence of God everywhere, as an all-pervasive, self-effulgent energy and consciousness.

This basic belief creates the attitude of sublime tolerance and acceptance toward others. Even tolerance is insufficient to describe the compassion and reverence the Hindu holds for the intrinsic sacredness within all things. Therefore, the actions of all Hindus are rendered benign, or *ahiṁsā*. One would not want to hurt something which one revered.

On the other hand, when the fundamentalists of any religion teach an unrelenting duality based on good and evil, man and nature or God and Devil, this creates friends and enemies. This belief is a sacrilege to Hindus, because they know that the attitudes which are the by-product are totally dualistic, and for good to triumph over that which is alien or evil, it must kill out that which is considered to be evil.

The Hindu looks at nothing as intrinsically evil. To him the ground is sacred. The sky is sacred. The sun is sacred. His wife is a Goddess. Her husband is a God. Their children are *devas*. Their home is a shrine. Life is a pilgrimage to *mukti*, or liberation from rebirth, which once attained is the end to reincarnation in a physical body. When on a holy pilgrimage, one would not want to hurt anyone along the way, knowing full well the experiences on this path are of one's own creation, though maybe acted out through others.

Noninjury for Renunciates

Ahiṁsā is the first and foremost virtue, presiding over truthfulness, nonstealing, sexual purity, patience, steadfastness, compassion, honesty and moderate appetite. The *brahmachārī* and *sannyāsin* must take *ahiṁsā*, noninjury, one step further. He has mutated himself, escalated himself, by stopping the abilities of being able to harm another by thought, word or deed, physically, mentally or emotionally. The one step further is that he must not harm his own self with his own thoughts, his own feelings, his own actions toward his own body, toward his own emotions, toward his own mind. This is very important to remember. And here, at this juncture, *ahiṁsā* has a tie with *satya,* truthfulness. The *sannyāsin* must be totally truthful to himself, to his *guru,* to the Gods and to Lord Śiva, who resides within him every minute of every hour of every day. But for him to truly know this and express it through his life and be a living religious example of the Sanātana Dharma, all tendencies toward *hiṁsā,* injuriousness, must always be definitely harnessed in chains of steel. The mystical reason is this. Because of the *brahmachārī's* or *sannyāsin's* spiritual power, he really has more ability to hurt someone than he or that person may know, and therefore his observance of noninjury is even more vital. Yes, this is true. A *brahmachārī* or *sannyāsin* who does not live the highest level of *ahiṁsā* is not a *brahmachārī.*

Words are expressions of thoughts, thoughts created from *prāṇa.* Words coupled with thoughts backed up by the transmuted *prāṇas,* or the accumulated bank account of energies held back within the *brahmachārī* and the *sannyāsin,* become powerful thoughts, and when expressed through words go deep into the mind, creating impressions, *saṁskāras,* that last a long time, maybe forever. It is truly unfortunate if a *brahmachārī* or *sannyāsin* loses control of himself and betrays *ahiṁsā* by becoming *hiṁsā,* an injurious person—unfortunate for those involved, but more unfortunate for himself. When we hurt another, we scar the inside of ourself; we clone the image. The scar would never leave the *sannyāsin* until it left the person that he hurt. This is because the *prāṇas,* the transmuted energies, give so much force to the thought. Thus the words penetrate to the very core of the being. Therefore, angry people should get married and should not practice *brahmacharya.*

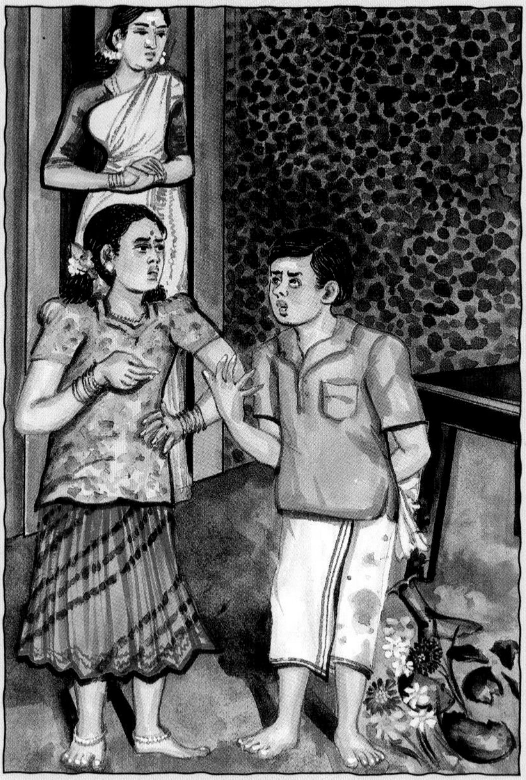

A boy has broken a vase and is denying the mischief. Mother watches, hoping he will learn to tell the truth.

Summary of the Second Restraint

Adhere to truthfulness, refraining from lying and betraying promises. Speak only that which is true, kind, helpful and necessary. Knowing that deception creates distance, don't keep secrets from family or loved ones. Be fair, accurate and frank in discussions, a stranger to deceit. Admit your failings. Do not engage in slander, gossip or backbiting. Do not bear false witness against another.

THE SECOND RESTRAINT

Truthfulness

Satya सत्य

S*ATYA*, TRUTHFULNESS, IS THE SECOND *YAMA*. IT SEEMS THAT LITTLE CHILDREN ARE NATURALLY TRUTHFUL, OPEN AND HONEST. THEIR LIVES ARE UNCOMPLICATED, AND THEY have no secrets. National studies show that children, even at an early age, learn to lie from their parents. They are taught to keep family secrets, whom to like, whom to dislike, whom to hate and whom to love, right within the home itself. Their minds become complicated and their judgments of what to say and what not to say are often influenced by the possibility of a punishment, perhaps a beating. Therefore, to fully encompass *satya* and incorporate it in one's life as a teenager or an adult, it is quite necessary to dredge the subconscious mind and in some cases reject much of what mother or father, relatives and elders had placed into it at an early age. Only by rejecting the apparent opposites, likes and dislikes, hates and loves, can true truthfulness, which is a quality of the soul, burst forth again and be there in full force as it is within an innocent child. A child practices truthfulness without wisdom. Wisdom, which is the timely application of knowledge, guides truthfulness for the adult. To attain wisdom, the adult must be conversant with the soul nature.

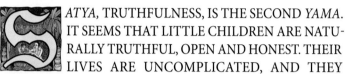

What is it that keeps us from practicing truthfulness? Fear, mainly. Fear of discovery, fear of punishment or loss of status. This is the most honest untruthfulness. The next layer of untruthfulness would be the mischievous person willing to take a chance of not being caught and deliberately inventing stories about another, deliberately lying when the truth would do just as well. The third and worst layer is calculated deception and breaking of promises.

Satya is a restraint, and as one of the ten restraints it ranks in importance as number two. When we restrain our tendencies to deceive, to lie and break promises, our external life is uncomplicated, as is our subconscious mind. Honesty is the foundation of truth. It is ecologically, psychologically purifying. However, many people are not truthful with themselves, to themselves, let alone to others. And the calculated, subconscious built-in program of these clever, cunning, two-faced individuals keeps them in the inner worlds of darkness. To emerge from those worlds, the practice of truthfulness, *satya,* is in itself a healing and purifying *sādhana.*

What is breaking a promise? Breaking a promise is, for example, when someone confides in you, asks you to keep it to yourself and not to tell anyone, and then you tell. You have betrayed your promise. Confidences must be kept at all costs in the practice of *satya.*

There are certainly times when withholding the truth is permitted. The *Tirukural, Weaver's Wisdom,* explains that "Even falsehood is of the nature of truth if it renders good results, free from fault" (292). An astrologer, for instance, while reviewing a chart would refrain from telling of a heartbreak that might come to a person at a certain time in his life. This is wisdom. In fact, astrologers are admonished by their *gurus* to hold back information that might be harmful or deeply discouraging. A doctor might not tell his patient that he will die in three days when he sees the vital signs weakening. Instead, he may encourage positive thinking, give hope, knowing that life is eternal and that to invoke fear might create depression and hopelessness in the mind of the ill person.

When pure truthfulness would injure or cause harm, then the first *yama, ahiṁsā,* would come into effect. You would not want to harm that person, even with the truth. But we must not look at this verse from the *Tirukural* as giving permission for deception. The spirit of the verse is wisdom, good judgment, not the subterfuge of telling someone you are going to Mumbai when your actual destination is Kalikot. That is not truthful. It would be much better to avoid answering the question at all in some way if one wanted to conceal the destination of his journey. This would be wisdom. You would not complicate your own subconscious mind by telling an untruth, nor be labeled deceptive in the mind of the informed person when he eventually discovers the actual truth.

Honesty with Your Guru

Some people use the excuse of truthfulness to nag their spouse about what they don't like about him or her, or to gossip about other people's flaws. This is not the spirit of *satya.* We do not want to expose others' faults. Such confrontations could become argumentative and combative. No one knows one's faults better than oneself. But fear and weakness often prevail, while motivation and a clear plan to correct the situation are absent. Therefore, to give a clear plan, a positive outlook, a new way of thinking, diverts the attention of the individual and allows internal healing to take place. This is wisdom. This is *ahiṁsā,* noninjury. This is *satya,* truthfulness. The wise devotee is careful to never insult or humiliate others, even under the pretext of telling the truth, which is an excuse that people sometimes use to tell others what they don't like about them. Wise devotees realize that there is good and bad in everyone. There are emotional ups and downs, mental elations and depressions, encouragements and discouragements. Let's focus on the positive. This is *ahiṁsā* and *satya* working together.

The *brahmachārī* and the *sannyāsin* must be absolutely truthful with their *satguru.* They must be absolutely diplomatic, wise and always accentuate the good qualities within the *sannyāsin* and *brahmachārī* communities. The *guru* has the right to discuss, rebuke or discipline the uncomely qualities in raising up the *brahmachārī* and *sannyāsin.* Only he has this right, because it was given to him by the *brahmachārīs* and *sannyāsins* when they took him as their *satguru.* This means that *brahmachārīs* and *sannyāsins* cannot discipline one another, psychoanalyze and correct in the name of truthfulness, without violation of the number one *yama—ahiṁsā,* noninjury.

Mothers and fathers have rights with their own children, as do *gurus* with their *śishyas.* These rights are limited according to wisdom. They are not all-inclusive and should not inhibit free will and well-rounded growth within an individual. This is why a *guru* is looked upon as the mother and father by the mother and father and by the disciple who is sent to the *guru's āśrama* to study and learn. It is the *guru*'s responsibility to mold the aspirant into a solid member of the monastic community, just as it is the mother's and father's duty to mold the youth to be a responsible, looked-up-to member of the family community. This is how society progresses.

The practice, *niyama,* to strengthen one's *satya* qualities is *tapas,* austerity—performing *sādhana,* penance, *tapas* and sacrifice. If you find you have not been truthful, if you have betrayed promises, then put yourself under the *tapas sādhana.* Perform a lengthy penance. Atone, repent, perform austerities. You will soon find that being truthful is much easier than what *tapas* and austerities will make you go through if you fail to restrain yourself.

Truthfulness is the fullness of truth. Truth itself is fullness. May fullness prevail, truth prevail, and the spirit of *satya* and *ahiṁsā* permeate humanity.

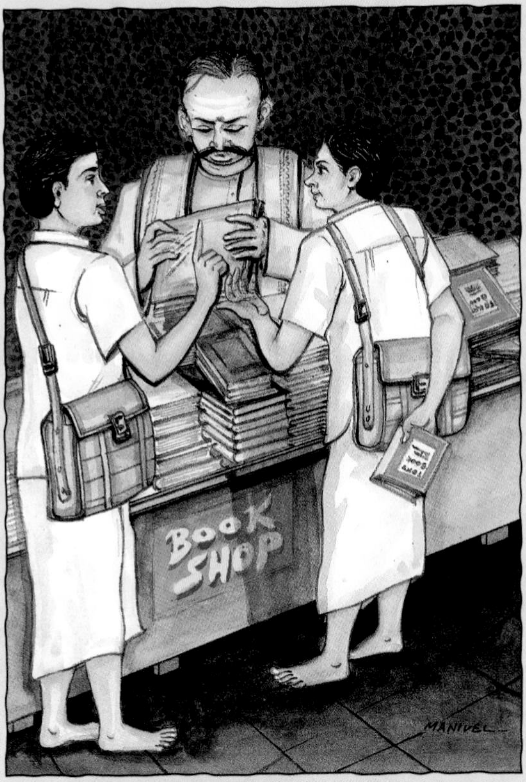

Two boys conspire to break the principle of asteya *as one distracts a merchant while the other steals a book.*

Summary of the Third Restraint

Uphold the virtue of nonstealing, neither thieving, coveting nor failing to repay debt. Control your desires and live within your means. Do not use borrowed resources for unintended purposes or keep them past due. Do not gamble or defraud others. Do not renege on promises. Do not use others' names, words, resources or rights without permission and acknowledgement.

THE THIRD RESTRAINT

Nonstealing

Asteya अस्तेय

A*STEYA* IS THE THIRD *YAMA*, NEITHER STEALING, NOR COVETING NOR ENTERING INTO DEBT. WE ALL KNOW WHAT STEALING IS. BUT NOW LET'S DEFINE COVETOUSNESS. IT could well be defined as owning something mentally and emotionally but not actually owning it physically. This is not good. It puts a hidden psychological strain on all parties concerned and brings up the lower emotions from the *tala chakras.* It must be avoided at all cost. Coveting is desiring things that are not your own. Coveting leads to jealousy, and it leads to stealing. The first impulse toward stealing is coveting, wanting. If you can control the impulse to covet, then you will not steal. Coveting is mental stealing.

Of course, stealing must never ever happen. Even a penny, a peso, a rupee, a lira or a yen should not be misappropriated or stolen. Defaulting on debts is also a form of stealing. But avoiding debt in principle does not mean that one cannot buy things on credit or through other contractual arrangements. It does mean that payments must be made at the expected time, that credit be given in trust and be eliminated when the time has expired, that contracts be honored to the satisfaction of all parties concerned. Running one's affairs on other peoples' money must be restrained. To control this is the *sādhana* of *asteya. Brahmachārīs* and *sannyāsins,* of course, must scrupulously obey these restraints relating to debt, stealing and covetousness. These are certainly not in their code of living.

To perfect *asteya,* we must practice *dāna,* charity, the third *niyama*; we must take the *dāśama bhāga vrata,* promising to tithe, pay *dāśamāṁśa,* to our favorite religious organization and, on top of that, give creatively, without thought of reward. Stealing is selfishness. Giving is unselfishness. Any lapse of *asteya* is corrected by *dāna.*

It is important to realize that one cannot simply obey the *yamas* without actively practicing the *niyamas.* To restrain one's current tendencies successfully, each must be replaced by a positive observance. For each of the *yamas,* there is a positive replacement of doing something else. The *niyamas* must totally overshadow the qualities controlled by the *yamas* for the perfect person to emerge. It is also important to remember that doing what should not be done—and not doing what should be done—does have its consequences. These can be many, depending upon the evolution of the soul of each individual; but all such acts bring about the lowering of consciousness into the instinctive nature, and inevitable suffering is the result. Each Hindu *guru* has his own ways of mitigating the negative *karmas* that result as a consequence of not living up to the high ideals of these precepts. But the world is also a *guru,* in a sense, and its devotees learn by their own mistakes, often repeating the same lessons many, many times.

Debt, Gambling and Grief

I was asked, "Is borrowing money to finance one's business in accord with the *yama* of nonstealing? When can you use other peoples' money and when should you not?" When the creditors start calling you for their money back, sending demand notices indicating that they only extended you thirty days', sixty days' or ninety days' credit, then if you fail to pay, or pay only a quarter or half of it just to keep them at arm's length because you still need their money to keep doing what you are doing, this is a violation of this *yama.*

There are several kinds of debt that are disallowed by this *yama.* One is spending beyond your means and accumulating bills you can't pay. We are reminded of *Tirukural* verse 478 which says that the way to avoid poverty is to spend within your means: "A small income is no cause for failure, provided expenditures do not exceed it." We can see that false wealth, or the mere appearance of wealth, is using other peoples' money, either against their will or by paying a premium price for it. Many people today are addicted to abusing credit. It's like being addicted to the drug opium. People addicted to O.P.M.—other people's money—compulsively spend beyond their means. They don't even think twice about handing over their last credit card to pay for that $500 *sārī* after all the other credit cards have been "maxed out." When the bill arrives, it gets added to the stack of other bills that can't possibly be paid.

Another kind of debt is contracting resources beyond your ability to pay back the loan. This is depending on a frail, uncertain future. Opportunities may occur to pay the debt, but then again they may not. The desire was so great for the commodity which caused the debt that a chance was taken. Essentially, this is gambling with someone else's money; and it is no way to run one's life.

Gambling and speculation are also forms of entering into debt. Speculation could be a proper form of acquiring wealth if one has the wealth to maintain the same standard of living he is accustomed to even if the speculation failed. Much of business is speculation; and high-risk speculations do come along occasionally; but one should never risk more than one can afford to lose.

Gambling is different, because the games are fun, a means of entertainment and releasing stress; though even in the casinos one should not gamble more than he could afford to lose. However, unlike speculation, when one is in the excitement of gambling and begins to lose, the greed and desire to win it all back arises, and the flustered gambler may risk his and his family's wealth and well-being.

Stress builds. The disastrous consequences of gambling were admonished in the oldest scripture, the *Ṛig Veda*, in the famous fourteen-verse "Gambler's Lament" (10.34. VE, P. 501). Verse ten summarizes: "Abandoned, the wife of the gambler grieves. Grieved, too, is his mother, as he wanders vaguely. Afraid and in debt, ever greedy for money, he steals in the night to the home of another." This is not fun; nor is it entertainment.

These are the grave concerns behind our *sūtra* in *Living with Śiva* that prohibits gambling for my *śishyas:* "Śiva's devotees are forbidden to indulge in gambling or games of chance with payment or risk, even through others or for employment. Gambling erodes society, assuring the loss of many for the gain of a few" *(sūtra* 76). Everyone really knows that the secret to winning at gambling is to own a casino.

Compulsive gambling and reckless, unfounded speculation are like stealing from your own family, risking the family wealth. More than that, it is stealing from yourself, because the remorse felt when an inevitable loss comes could cause a loss of faith in your abilities and your judgment. And if the loss affects the other members of the family, their estimation and respect and confidence in your good judgment goes way down.

Many people justify stealing by saying that life is unfair and therefore it's OK to take from the rich. They feel it's OK to steal from a rich corporation, for example: "They will never miss it, and we need it more." Financial speculation can easily slide into unfair maneuvering, where a person is actually stealing from a small or large company, thereby making it fail. The credibility of the person will go down, and businesses will beware of this speculative investor who would bring a company to ruin to fatten his own pockets. Entering into debt is a modern convenience and a modern temptation. But this convenience must be honored within the time allotted. If you are paying a higher interest rate because of late or partial payments, you have abused your credit and your creditors.

At the Global Forum for Human Survival in 1990 in Moscow, the participants began worrying about the kids, the next generation. "What are they going to think of us?" they asked. Is it fair to fulfill a need now, spoil the environment and hand the bill over to the next generation? No, it is not. This is another form of stealing. We can't say, "We have to have chlorofluorocarbons now, and the next generation has to face the consequences." The *yamas* and *niyamas* are thus not just a personal matter but also a national, communal and global matter. Yes, this takes *asteya* and all the restraints and observances to another dimension.

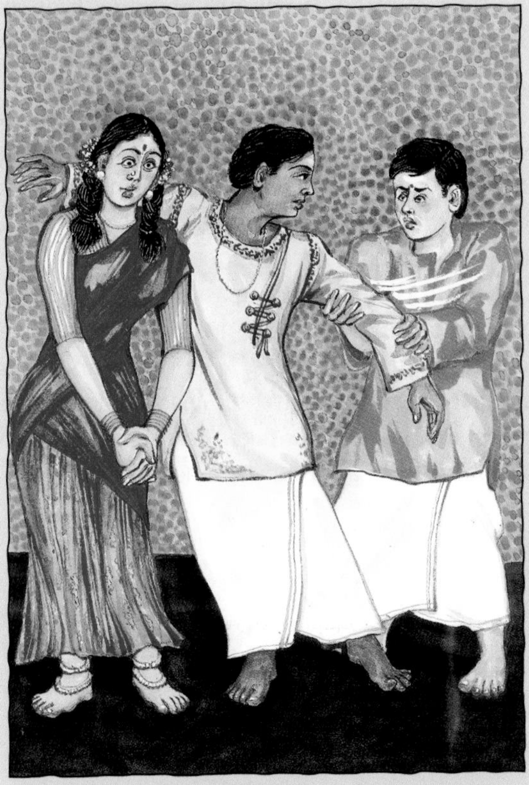

A brother guards his sister's purity, brahmacharya, *from a rogue who has approached her immodestly.*

❁

Summary of the Fourth Restraint

Practice divine conduct, controlling lust by remaining celibate when single and faithful in marriage. Before marriage, use vital energies in study, and after marriage in creating family success. Don't waste the sacred force by promiscuity in thought, word or deed. Be restrained with the opposite sex. Seek holy company. Dress and speak modestly. Shun pornography, sexual humor and violence.

THE FOURTH RESTRAINT

Sexual Purity

Brahmacharya ब्रह्मचर्य

BRAHMACHARYA, SEXUAL PURITY, IS A VERY IMPORTANT RESTRAINT AMONG THE ANCIENT ŚAIVITE ETHICAL PRINCIPLES KNOWN AS *YAMAS* AND *NIYAMAS*, BECAUSE IT SETS the pattern for one's entire life. Following this principle, the vital energies are used before marriage in study rather than in sexual fantasy, e-pornography, masturbation, necking, petting or sexual intercourse. After marriage, the vital energies are concentrated on business, livelihood, fulfilling one's duties, serving the community, improving oneself and one's family, and performing *sādhana*. For those who do not believe in God, Gods, *guru* or the path to enlightenment, this is a difficult restraint to fulfill, and such people tend to be promiscuous when single and therefore unfaithful in marriage.

The rewards for maintaining this restraint are many. Those who practice *brahmacharya* before marriage and apply its principles throughout married life are free from encumbrances—mentally, emotionally and physically. They get a good start on life, have long-lasting, mature family relationships, and their children are emotionally sound, mentally firm and physically strong.

Those who are promiscuous and unreligious are susceptible to impulses of anger, have undefined fears, experience jealousy and the other instinctive emotions. The doors of the higher world are open to them, but the doors of the lower world are also open. Even the virgin *brahmachārī* who believes firmly in God, Gods, *guru* and the path to enlightenment and has a strict family must be watched and carefully guided to maintain his *brahmacharya.* Without this careful attention, the virginity may easily be lost.

Brahmacharya for the monastic means complete sexual abstinence and is, of course, an understood requirement to maintain this position in life. This applies as well to any single individual who has taken the celibacy vow, known as *brahmacharya vrata.* If *brahmacharya* is compromised by the *brahmachārī,* he must face the consequences and reaffirm his original intent. Having lost faith in himself because of breaking his *vrata,* his self-confidence must be rebuilt.

It should be perfectly clear that it is totally unacceptable for men or women who have taken up the celibate monastic life to live a double standard and surround themselves with those of the opposite sex—be they fellow *āśramites,* personal aides, secretaries or close devotees—or with their former family. Nowadays there are *pseudo-sannyāsins* who are married and call themselves *swāmīs,* but, if pressed, they might admit that they are simply *yoga* teachers dressed in orange robes, bearing the title "*swāmī*" to attract the attention of the uninformed public for commercial reasons.

There is great power in the practice of *brahmacharya,* literally "Godly conduct." Containing the sacred fluids within the body builds up a bank account through the years that makes the realization of God on the path to enlightenment a reality within the life of the individual who is single. When *brahmacharya* is broken through sexual intercourse, this power goes away. It just goes away.

Brahmacharya in Family Life

The observance of *brahmacharya* is perhaps the most essential aspect of a sound, spiritual culture. This is why in Śaivism boys and girls are taught the importance of remaining celibate until they are married. This creates healthy individuals, physically, emotionally and spiritually, generation after generation. There is a mystical reason. In virgin boys and girls, the psychic *nāḍīs*, the astral nerve currents that extend out into and through their aura, have small hooks at the end. When a boy and girl marry, the hooks straighten out and the *nāḍīs* are tied one to another, and they actually grow together. If the first sexual experience is premarital and virginity is broken, the hooks at the end of the *nāḍīs* also straighten out, but there is nothing to grow onto if the partners do not marry. Then, when either partner marries someone else, the relationship is never as close as when a virgin boy and girl marry, because their *nāḍīs* don't grow together in the same way. In cases such as this, they feel the need for intellectual stimuli and emotional stimuli to keep the marriage going.

Youth ask, "How should we regard members of the opposite sex?" Do not look at members of the opposite sex with any idea of sex or lust in mind. Do not indulge in admiring those of the opposite sex, or seeing one as more beautiful than another. Boys must foster the inner attitude that all young women are their sisters and all older women are their mother. Girls must foster the inner attitude that all young men are their brothers and all older men are their father. Do not attend movies that depict the base instincts of humans, nor read books or magazines of this nature. Above all, avoid pornography on the Internet, on TV and in any other media.

To be successful in *brahmacharya,* one naturally wants to avoid arousing the sex instincts. This is done by understanding and avoiding the eight successive phases: fantasy, glorification, flirtation, lustful glances, secret love talk, amorous longing, rendezvous and finally intercourse. Be very careful to mix only with good company—those who think and speak in a cultured way—so that the mind and emotions are not led astray and vital energies needed for study used up. Get plenty of physical exercise. This is very important, because exercise sublimates your instinctive drives and directs excess energy and the flow of blood into all parts of the body.

Brahmacharya means sexual continence, as was observed by Mahatma Gandhi in his later years and by other great souls throughout life. There is another form of sexual purity, though not truly *brahmacharya*, followed by faithful family people who have a normal sex life while raising a family. They are working toward the stage when they will take their *brahmacharya vrata* after sixty years of age. Thereafter they would live together as brother and sister, sleeping in separate bedrooms. During their married life, they control the forces of lust and regulate instinctive energies and thus prepare to take that *vrata*. But if they are unfaithful, flirtatious and loose in their thinking through life, they will not be inclined to take the *vrata* in later life.

Faithfulness in marriage means fidelity and much more. It includes mental faithfulness, non-flirtatiousness and modesty toward the opposite sex. A married man, for instance, should not hire a secretary who is more magnetic or more beautiful than his wife. Metaphysically, in the perfect family relationship, man and wife are, in a sense, creating a one nervous system for their joint spiritual progress, and all of their *nāḍīs* are growing together over the years. If they break that faithfulness, they break the psychic, soul connections that are developing for their personal inner achievements. If one or the other of the partners does have an affair, this creates a psychic tug and pull on the nerve system of both spouses that will continue until the affair ends and long afterwards. Therefore, the principle of the containment of the sexual force and mental and emotional impulses is the spirit of *brahmacharya*, both for the single and married person.

Rules for Serious People

For virtuous individuals who marry, their experiences with their partner are, again, free from lustful fantasies; and emotional involvement is only with their spouse. Yes, a normal sex life should be had between husband and wife, and no one else should be included in either one's mind or emotions. Never hugging, touching another's spouse or exciting the emotions; always dressing modestly, not in a sexually arousing way; not viewing sexually oriented or pornographic videos; not telling dirty jokes—all of these simple customs are traditional ways of upholding sexual purity. The *yama* of *brahmacharya* works in concert with *asteya,* nonstealing. Stealing or coveting another's spouse, even mentally, creates a force that, once generated, is difficult to stop.

In this day and age, when promiscuity is a way of life, there is great strength in married couples' understanding and applying the principles of sexual purity. If they obey these principles and are on the path of enlightenment, they will again become celibate later in life, as they were when they were young. These principles persist through life, and when their children are raised and the forces naturally become quiet, around age sixty, husband and wife take the *brahmacharya vrata,* live in separate rooms and prepare themselves for greater spiritual experiences.

Married persons uphold sexual purity by observing the eightfold celibacy toward everyone but their spouse. These are ideals for serious, spiritual people. For those who have nothing to do with spirituality, these laws are meaningless. We are assuming a situation of a couple where everything they do and all that happens in their life is oriented toward spiritual life and spiritual goals and, therefore, these principles do apply. For sexual purity, individuals must believe firmly in the path to enlightenment. They must have faith in higher powers than themselves. Without this, sexual purity is nearly impossible.

One of the fastest ways to destroy the stability of families and societies is through promiscuity, mental and/or physical, and the best way to maintain stability is through self-control. The world today has become increasingly unstable because of the mental, physical, emotional license that people have given to themselves. The generation that follows an era of promiscuity has a dearth of examples to follow and are even more unstable than their parents were when they began their promiscuous living. Stability for human society is based on morality, and morality is based on harnessing and controlling sexuality. The principles of *brahmacharya* should be learned well before puberty, so that the sexual feelings the young person then begins to experience are free of mental fantasies and emotional involvement. Once established in a young person, this control is expected to be carried out all through life. When a virgin boy and girl marry, they transfer the love they have for their parents to one another. The boy's attachment to his mother is transferred to his wife, and the girl's attachment to her father is transferred to her husband. She now becomes the mother. He now becomes the father. This does not mean they love their parents any less. This is why the parents have to be in good shape, to create the next generation of stable families. This is their *dharmic* duty. If they don't do it, they create all kinds of uncomely *karmas* for themselves to be faced at a later time.

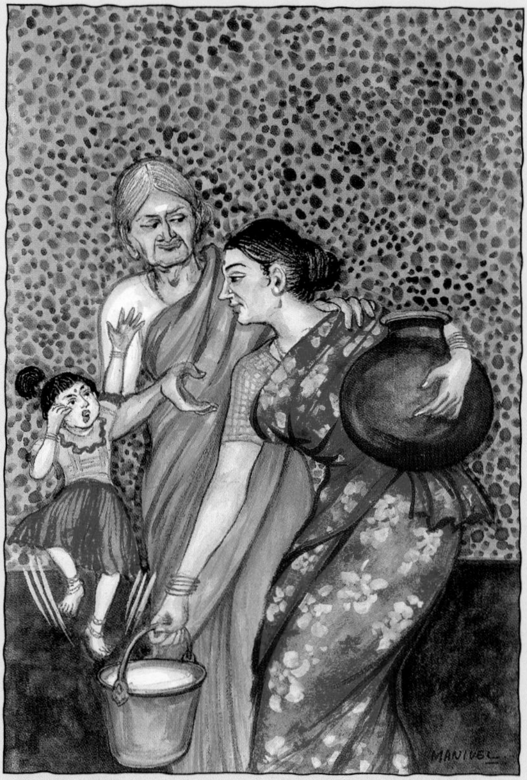

Kshamā *is epitomized by a mother's patiently setting aside her urgent duties to tend to her daugher's tears.*

❁

Summary of the Fifth Restraint

Exercise patience, restraining intolerance with people and impatience with circumstances. Be agreeable. Let others behave according to their nature, without adjusting to you. Don't argue, dominate conversations or interrupt others. Don't be in a hurry. Be patient with children and the elderly. Minimize stress by keeping worries at bay. Remain poised in good times and bad.

THE FIFTH RESTRAINT

Patience

Kshamā क्षमा

PATIENCE, OR *KSHAMĀ*, THE FIFTH *YAMA*, IS AS ESSENTIAL TO THE SPIRITUAL PATH AS THE SPIRITUAL PATH IS TO ITSELF. IMPATIENCE IS A SIGN OF DESIROUSNESS TO FULFILL UNFULfilled desires, having no time for any interruptions or delays from anything that seems irrelevant to what one really wants to accomplish.

We must restrain our desires by regulating our life with daily worship and meditation. Daily worship and meditation are difficult to accomplish without a break in continuity. However, impatience and frustration come automatically in continuity, day after day, often at the same time—being impatient before breakfast because it is not served on time, feeling intolerant and abusive with children because they are not behaving as adults, and on and on. Everything has its timing and its regularity in life. Focusing on living in the eternity of the moment overcomes impatience. It produces the feeling that one has nothing to do, no future to work toward and no past to rely on. This excellent spiritual practice can be performed now and again during the day by anyone.

Patience is having the power of acceptance, accepting people, accepting events as they are happening. One of the great spiritual powers that people can have is to accept things as they are. That forestalls impatience and intolerance. Acceptance is developed in a person by understanding the law of *karma* and in seeing God Śiva and His work everywhere, accepting the perfection of the timing of the creation, preservation and absorption of the entire universe.

Acceptance does not mean being resigned to one's situation and avoiding challenges. We know that we ourselves created our own situation, our own challenges, in a former time by sending forth our energies, thoughts, words and deeds. As these energies, on their cycle-back, manifest through people, happenings and circumstances, we must patiently deal with the situation, not fight it or try to avoid it or be discouraged because of it. This is *kshamā* in the raw. This is pure *kshamā*. Patience cannot be acquired in depth in any other way. This is why meditation upon the truths of the Sanātana Dharma is so important.

It is also extremely important to maintain patience with oneself—especially with oneself. Many people are masters of the façade of being patient with others but take their frustrations out on themselves. This can be corrected and must be corrected for spiritual unfoldment to continue through an unbroken routine of daily worship and meditation and a yearly routine of attending festivals and of pilgrimage, *tīrthayatra*.

Most people today are intolerant with one another and impatient with their circumstances. This breeds an irreverent attitude. Nothing is sacred to them, nothing holy. But through daily exercising anger, malice and the other lower emotions, they do, without knowing, invoke the demonic forces of the Narakaloka. Then they must suffer the backlash: have nightmares, confusions, separations and even perform heinous acts. Let all people of the world restrain themselves and be patient through the practice of daily worship and meditation, which retroactively invokes the divine forces from the Devaloka. May a great peace pervade the planet as the well-earned result of these practices.

The next time you find yourself becoming impatient, just stop for a moment and remember that you are on the upward path, now facing a rare opportunity to take one more step upward by overcoming these feelings, putting all that you have previously learned into practice. One does not progress on the spiritual path by words, ideas or unused knowledge. Memorized precepts, *ślokas,* all the shoulds and should-nots, are good, but unless used they will not propel you one inch further than you already are. It is putting what you have learned into practice in these moments of experiencing impatience and controlling it through command of your spiritual will, that moves you forward. These steps forward can never be retracted. When a test comes, prevail.

Sādhakas and *sannyāsins* must be perfect in *kshamā,* forbearing with people and patient under all circumstances, as they have harnessed their *karmas* of this life and the lives before, compressed them to be experienced in this one lifetime. There is no cause for them, if they are to succeed, to harbor intolerance or experience any kind of impatience with people or circumstances. Their instinctive, intellectual nature should be caught up in daily devotion, unreserved worship, meditation and deep self-inquiry. Therefore, the practice, *niyama,* that mitigates intolerance is devotion, Īśvarapūjana, cultivating devotion through daily worship and meditation.

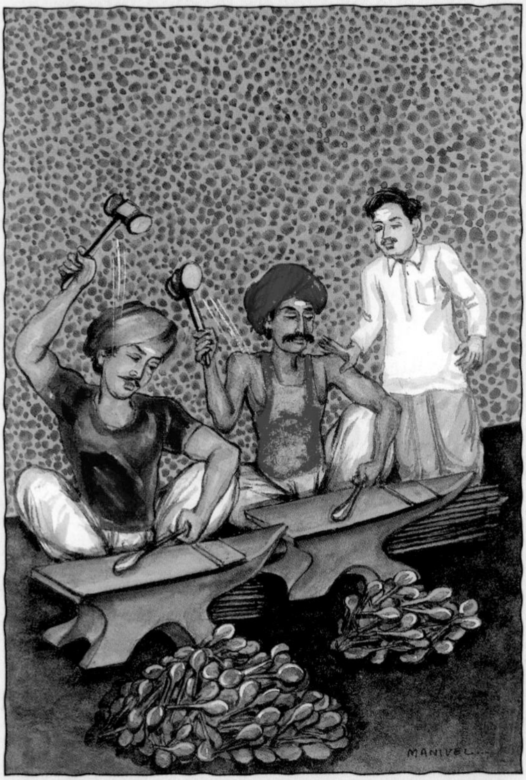

The worker on the left works steadily and energetically, exemplifying dhṛiti, *while the other is less productive.*

Summary of the Sixth Restraint

Foster steadfastness, overcoming nonperseverance, fear, indecision and changeableness. Achieve your goals with a prayer, purpose, plan, persistence and push. Be firm in your decisions. Avoid sloth and procrastination. Develop willpower, courage and industriousness. Overcome obstacles. Never carp or complain. Do not let opposition or fear of failure result in changing strategies.

THE SIXTH RESTRAINT

Steadfastness

Dhṛiti धृति

STEADFASTNESS, *DHṚITI,* IS THE SIXTH *YAMA.* TO BE STEADFAST, YOU HAVE TO USE YOUR WILLPOWER. WILLPOWER IS DEVELOPED EASILY IN A PERSON WHO HAS AN ADEQUATE memory and good reasoning faculties. To be steadfast as we go through life, we must have a purpose, a plan, persistence and push. Then nothing is impossible within the circumference of our *prārabdha karma*s.

It is impossible to be steadfast if we are not obeying the other restraints that the *ṛishis* of the Himalayas laid down for us as the fruits of their wisdom. All of these restraints build character, and *dhṛiti,* steadfastness, rests on the foundation of good character. Character—the ability to "act with care"—is built slowly, over time, with the help of relatives, preceptors and good-hearted friends. Observe those who are steadfast. You will learn from them. Observe those who are not, and they, too, will teach you. They will teach what you should not do. To be indecisive and changeable is not how we should be on the path to enlightenment, nor to be successful in any other pursuit. Nonperseverance and fear must be overcome, and much effort is required to accomplish this. Daily *sādhana,* preferably under a *guru's* guidance, is suggested here to develop a spiritual will and intellect.

In the *Śāndilya Upanishad, dhṛiti* has been described as preserving firmness of mind during the period of gain or loss of relatives. This implies that during times of sorrow, difficult *karmas,* loss and temptation, when in mental pain and anguish, feeling alone and neglected, we can persevere, be decisive and bring forth the *dhṛiti* strength within us and thus prevail. One translator of the *Varuha Upanishad* used the word *courage* to translate *dhṛiti*. Courageous and fearless people who are just and honest prevail over all *karmas*—benevolent, terrible and confused. This virtue is much like the monk's vow of humility, part of which is enduring hardship with equanimity, ease of mind, which means not panicking. The *Tirukural* reminds us, "It is the nature of asceticism to patiently endure hardship and to not harm living creatures" (261). And we can say that *dhṛiti* itself is a "hard ship"—a ship that can endure and persevere on its course even when tossed about on the waves of a turbulent sea.

Some might wonder why it is good to passively endure hardship. To persevere through hardship one must understand, as all Hindus do, that any hardship coming to us we ourselves participated in setting into motion in the past. To endure hardship and rise above it in consciousness is to overcome that *karma* forever. To resent hardship, to fight it, is to have it return later at a most inconvenient time.

An essential part of steadfastness is overcoming changeableness. Changeableness means indecision, not being decisive, changing one's mind after making a deliberate, positive decision. Changing one's mind can be a positive thing, but making a firm, well-considered decision and not following it through would gain one the reputation of not being dependable, even of being weak-minded. No one wants a reputation like this.

How can we discriminate between this and the strength of a person who changes his or her mind in wisdom because of changes of circumstance? A person who is changeable is fickle and unsure of himself, changing without purpose or reason. *Dhṛiti*, steadfastness, describes the mind that is willing to change for mature reasons based on new information but holds steady to its determinations through thick and thin in the absence of such good reasons. Its decisions are based on wise discrimination. A person who is patient and truthful, who would not harm others by thought, word or deed and who is compassionate and honest has the strong nature of one who is firm in *dhṛiti,* steadfastness. He is the prevailer over obstacles. One firm in *dhṛiti* can be leaned upon by others, depended upon. He is charitable, has faith in God, Gods and *guru,* worships daily and manifests in his life a spiritual will and intellect. In relaxed moments he experiences *santosha,* contentment, not being preoccupied by feelings of responsibility, duty or things left undone.

The spiritual path is a long, enduring process. It does not reach fruition in a year or two years. The spiritual path brings lots of ups and downs, and the greatest challenges will come to the greatest souls. With this in mind, it becomes clear that steadiness and perseverance are absolutely essential on the spiritual path.

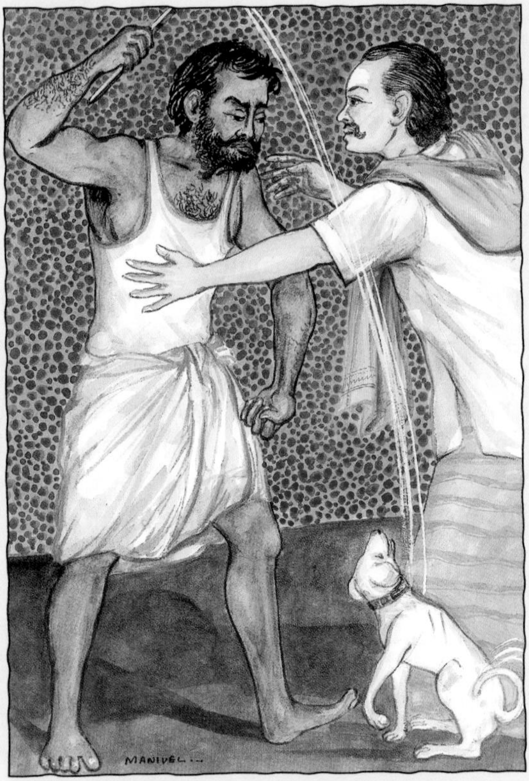

The man beating his dog has little compassion, dayā. *A friend urges him to cognize the cruelty of his actions.*

Summary of the Seventh Restraint

Practice compassion, conquering callous, cruel and insensitive feelings toward all beings. See God everywhere. Be kind to people, animals, plants and the Earth itself. Forgive those who apologize and show true remorse. Foster sympathy for others' needs and suffering. Honor and assist those who are weak, impoverished, aged or in pain. Oppose family abuse and other cruelties.

THE SEVENTH RESTRAINT

Compassion

Dayā दया

DAYĀ, COMPASSION, IS THE SEVENTH *YAMA*. SOMETIMES IT IS KIND TO BE CRUEL, AND AT OTHER TIMES IT IS CRUEL TO BE KIND. THIS STATEMENT HAS COME FORWARD FROM religion to religion, generation to generation. Compassion tempers all decisions, gives clemency, absolution, forgiveness as a boon even for the most heinous misdeeds. This is a quality built on steadfastness. *Dayā* comes from deep *sādhana,* prolonged *santosha,* contentment, scriptural study and listening to the wise. It is the outgrowth of the unfolded soul, the maturing of higher consciousness. A compassionate person transcends even forgiveness by caring for the suffering of the person he has forgiven. The compassionate person is like a God. He is the boon-giver. Boons, which are gifts from the Gods, come unexpectedly, unasked-for. And so it is with the grace of a compassionate person.

A devotee asked, "What should we think about those who are cruel toward creatures, who casually kill flies and step on cockroaches?" Compassion is defined as conquering callous, cruel and insensitive feelings toward all beings. A compassionate person would tell a plant verbally if he was going to pick from it, intuiting that the plant has feelings of its own. A compassionate person would seek to keep pests away rather than killing them. A callous person would tear the plant up by its roots. A cruel person would, as a child, pull one wing off a fly and, unless corrected, mature this cruelty on through life until he maimed a fellow human. Compassion is just the opposite to all this.

When we find callous, cruel and insensitive people in

our midst, we should not take them into our inner circles, but make them feel they must improve before admittance onto the spiritual path. Compassion is the outgrowth of being forgiving. It is the outgrowth of truthfulness, and of noninjury. It is a product of *asteya,* of *brahmacharya* and of *kshamā.* It is, in fact, higher consciousness, based in the *viśuddha chakra* of divine love.

One can't command compassion. Before compassion comes love. Compassion is the outgrowth of love. Love is the outgrowth of understanding. Understanding is the outgrowth of reason. One must have sufficient memory to remember the various points of reason and enough willpower to follow them through to be able to psychically look into the core of existence to gain the reverence for all life, all living organisms, animate or inanimate. Compassion is a very advanced spiritual quality. When you see it exhibited in someone, you know he is very advanced spiritually—probably an old soul. It really can't be taught. *Dayā* goes with *ānanda.* Compassion and bliss are a one big package.

What is the difference between *ahiṁsā* and *dayā,* compassion, one might ask? There is a distinct difference. Not harming others by thought, word or deed is a cardinal law of Hinduism and cannot be avoided, discarded, ignored or replaced by the more subtle concept of compassion. *Ahiṁsā,* among the *yamas* and *niyamas,* could be considered the only explicit commandment Hinduism gives. Compassion comes from the heart, comes spontaneously. It is a total flow of spiritual, material, intellectual giving, coming unbidden to the receiver.

Compassion by no means is foolishness or pretense. It is an overflowing of soulfulness. It is an outpouring of spiritual energy that comes through the person despite his thoughts or his personal feelings or his reason or good judgment. The person experiencing compassion is often turned around emotionally and mentally as he is giving this clemency, this boon of absolution, despite his own instinctive or intellectual inclinations. This is a spiritual outpouring through a person. Rishi Tirumular used the word *arul* for this *yama. Arul* means grace in the ancient Tamil language.

A devotee once e-mailed me, saying, "Recently I was going through some suffering and had bad thoughts and bad feelings for those who caused that suffering. Now that I'm feeling better, can I erase those bad thoughts and feelings?" Thoughts and bad feelings you have sent into the future are bound to come back to you. But, yes, you can mitigate and change that *karma* by being extra-special nice to those who abused you, hurt you or caused you to have bad thoughts and feelings against them. Being extra-special nice means accepting them for who they are. Don't have critical thoughts or try to change them. Have compassion. They are who they are, and only they can change themselves. Be extra-special nice. Go out of your way to say good words, give a gift and have good feelings toward them.

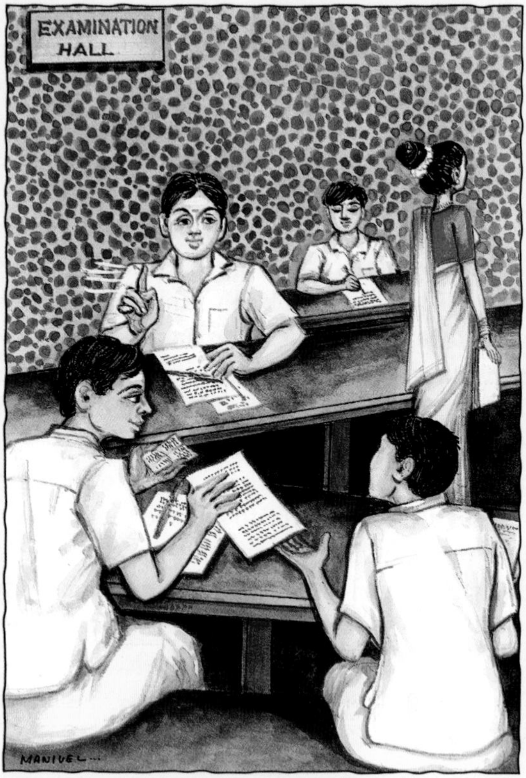

Two students are cheating on a test while a peer admonishes them to follow ārjava, *honesty.*

Summary of the Eighth Restraint

Maintain honesty, renouncing deception and wrongdoing. Act honorably even in hard times. Obey the laws of your nation and locale. Pay your taxes. Be straightforward in business. Do an honest day's work. Do not bribe or accept bribes. Do not cheat, deceive or circumvent to achieve an end. Be frank with yourself. Face and accept your faults without blaming them on others.

THE EIGHTH RESTRAINT

Honesty

Ārjava आर्जव

HONESTY, *ĀRJAVA*, IS THE EIGHTH *YAMA*. THE MOST IMPORTANT RULE OF HONESTY IS TO BE HONEST TO ONESELF, TO BE ABLE TO FACE UP TO OUR PROBLEMS AND ADMIT THAT WE have been the creator of them. To be able to then reason them through, make soulfully honest decisions toward their solutions, is a boon, a gift from the Gods. To be honest with oneself brings peace of mind. Those who are frustrated, discontent, are now and have been dishonest with themselves. They blame others for their own faults and predicaments. They are always looking for a scapegoat, someone to blame something on. To deceive oneself is truly the ultimate of wrongdoing. To deceive oneself is truly ignorance in its truest form. Honesty begins within one's own heart and soul and works its way out from there into dealing with other people. Polonius wisely said in Shakespeare's *Hamlet,* "This above all: to your own self be true, and it must follow, as the night the day, you cannot then be false to any man."

The adage, "Say what you mean, and mean what you say" should be heard again and again by the youth, middle-aged and elderly alike. Sir Walter Scott once said, "Oh what a tangled web we weave when first we practice to deceive." Mark Twain observed, "The advantage of telling the truth is that you don't have to remember what you said." Another philosopher, wise in human nature, noted, "You can watch a thief, but you cannot watch a liar." To be deceptive and not straightforward is thieving time from those you are deceiving. They are giving you their heart and mind, and you are twisting their thoughts to your own selfish ends, endeavoring to play them out, to take what they have, in favors or in kind, for your personal gain.

Deception is the cruelest of acts. A deceptive person is an insidious disease to society. Many parents, we are told, teach their children to be deceptive and cunning in order to get on in the world. They are not building good citizens. They are creating potential criminals who will eventually, if they perfect the art, ravage humankind. To be straightforward is the solution, no matter how difficult it is. To show remorse, be modest and show shame for misdeeds is the way to win back the faith, though maybe not the total trust, and a smidgen of respect from those who have discovered and exposed your deception. *Ārjava* is straightness with neighbors, family and with your government. You pay your taxes. You observe the laws. You don't fudge, bribe, cheat, steal or participate in fraud and other forms of manipulation.

Bribery corrupts the giver, the taker and the nation. It would be better not to have, not to do, and to live the simple life, if bribery were the alternative. To participate in bribery is to go into a deceptive, illegal partnership between the briber and the bribed. If and when discovered, embarrassment no end would fall on both parties involved in the crime, and even if not discovered, someone knows, someone is watching, your own conscience is watching. There is no law in any legal code of any government that says bribery is acceptable.

There are those who feel it is sufficient to be honest and straightforward with their friends and family, but feel justified to be dishonest with business associates, corporations, governments and strangers. These are the most despicable people. Obviously they have no knowledge of the laws of *karma* and no desire to obtain a better, or even a similar, birth. They may experience several abortions before obtaining a new physical body and then be an unwanted child. They may suffer child abuse, neglect, beatings, perhaps even be killed at a young age. These two-faced persons—honest to immediate friends and relatives, but dishonest and deceptive and involved in wrongdoings with business associates and in public life—deserve the punishment that only the lords of *karma* are able to deal out. These persons are training their sons and daughters to be like themselves and pull down humanity rather than uplift mankind.

Honesty in Monastic Life

We can say that *sādhakas, yogīs* and *swāmīs* upholding their vows are the prism of honesty. The rays of their auras radiate out through all areas of life. They are the protectors, the stabilizers, the uplifters, the consolers, the sympathizers. They have the solution to all human problems and all human ills, or they know where to find those solutions, to whom to go or what scripture to read. To be a *sādhaka, yogī* or *swāmī,* honesty is the primal qualification, yes, primal qualification—honesty, *ārjava.* No *satguru* would accept a monastic candidate who persists in patterns of deception, wrongdoing and outright lies and who shows no shame for misdeeds.

Human relations, especially the *guru*-disciple relationship, derive their strength from trust, which each shares and expresses. The breaking of the *yama* of *ārjava* is the severing of that trust, which thereby provokes the destruction or demise of the relationship. When the relationship falls into distrust, suspicion, anger, hate, confusion and retaliation, this gives birth to argument.

Countries that have weak leadership and unstable governments that allow wrongdoing to become a way of life, deception to be the way of thinking, are participating in dividing the masses in this very way. People begin to distrust one another. Because they are involved in wrongdoing, they suspect others of being involved in wrongdoings. People become angry because they are involved in wrongdoing. And finally the country fails and goes into war or succumbs to innumerable internal problems. We see this happening all over the world. A strong democratic country is constantly showing up politicians who take bribes and presidents who are involved in deception and wrongdoing, who set a poor example for the masses as to how things should be. Higher-consciousness governments are able to maintain their economy and feed their people. Lower-consciousness governments are not.

Even large, successful corporate monopolies deem honesty as the first necessary qualification for an employee. When his deception and wrongdoing are discovered, he is irrevocably terminated. There are many religious organizations today that have deceptive, dishonest people within them who connive wrongdoings, and these religious groups are failing and reaping the rewards of failing through loss and confusion. It is up to the heads of those organizations to weed out the deceptive, corruptive, virus-like persons to maintain the spirituality and fulfill the original intent of the founders.

Ārjava could well be interpreted as simplicity, as many commentators have done. It is easier to remember the truth than remember lies—white lies, gray lies or black lies. It is easier to be straightforward than conniving and deceptive, dishonest. A simple life is an honest life. An honest life is a simple life. When our wants which produce our needs are simple, there is no need to be deceptive or participate in wrongdoing. It's as simple as that. *Ārjava* means not complicating things, not ramifying concerns and anxieties. This is to say, when a situation occurs, handle the situation within the situation itself. Don't use the emotion involved in the situation to motivate or manipulate for personal gain in another situation. Don't owe people favors, and don't allow people to owe you favors. Don't promise what you can't deliver, and do deliver what you promise. This is the Sanātana Dharma way. If the neo-Indian religion is teaching differently, pay no attention. It is all political, and it has no kinship to *dharma*.

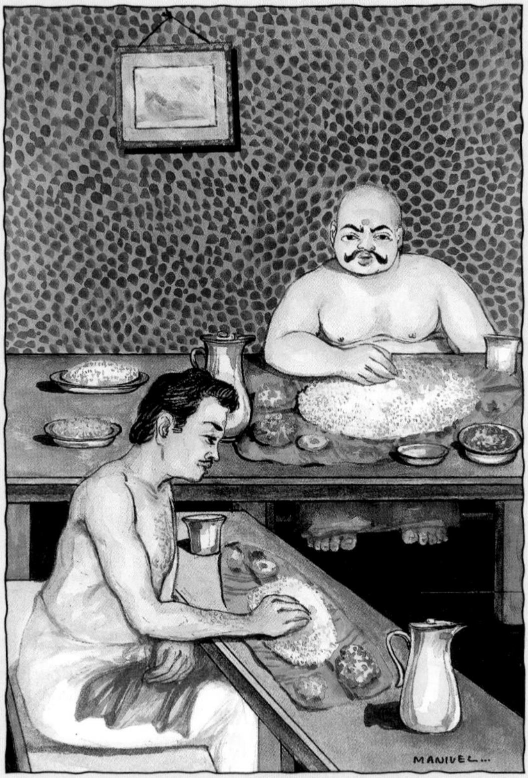

At a cafe two men enjoy a rice and curry meal on banana leaves. One follows mitāhāra, *while the other overeats.*

Summary of the Ninth Restraint

Be moderate in appetite, neither eating too much nor consuming meat, fish, shellfish, fowl or eggs. Enjoy fresh, wholesome vegetarian foods that vitalize the body. Avoid junk food. Drink in moderation. Eat at regular times, only when hungry, at a moderate pace, never between meals, in a disturbed atmosphere or when upset. Follow a simple diet, avoiding rich or fancy fare.

THE NINTH RESTRAINT

Moderate Diet

Mitāhara मिताहर

MITĀHĀRA, MODERATE APPETITE, IS THE TENTH *YAMA*. SIMILARLY, *MITAVYAYIN* IS LITTLE OR MODERATE SPENDING, BEING ECONOMICAL OR FRUGAL, AND *MITASĀYAN IS* is sleeping little. Gorging oneself has always been a form of decadence in every culture and is considered unacceptable behavior. It is the behavior of people who gain wealth and luxuries from the miseries of others. Decadence, which is a dance of decay, has been the downfall of many governments, empires, kingdoms and principalities. Marie Antoinette, Queen of France, made the famous decadent statement just before the French Revolution: "If the people have no bread, let them eat cake." Nearly everyone who heard that imperious insult, including its authoress, completely lost their heads. Decadence is a form of decay that the masses have railed against century upon century, millennium after millennium.

All this and more shows us that *mitāhāra* is a restraint that we must all obey and which is one of the most difficult. The body knows no wisdom as to shoulds and should-nots. It would eat and drink itself to death if it had its way, given its own instinctive intelligence. It is the mind that controls the body and emotions and must effect this restraint for its own preservation, health and wellness of being, to avoid the emptiness of "sick-being."

According to *āyurveda,* not eating too much is the greatest thing you can do for health if you want a long life, ease in meditation and a balanced, happy mind. That is why, for thousands of years, *yogīs, sādhus* and meditators have eaten moderately. There is almost nothing, apart from smoking and drugs, that hurts the body more than excessive eating, and excessive eating has to be defined in both the amount of food and the quality of food. If you are regularly eating rich, processed, dead foods, then you are not following *mitāhāra*, and you will have rich, finely processed, dead, dredged-up-from-the-past *karmic* experiences that will ruin your marriage, wreak havoc on your children and send you early to the funeral pyre.

For the twenty-first century, *mitāhāra* has still another meaning. Our *ṛishis* may have anticipated that the economy of *mitāhāra* makes it a global discipline—eating frugally, not squandering your wealth to overindulge yourself, not using the wealth of a nation to pamper the nation's most prosperous, not using the resources of the Earth to satiate excessive appetites. If all are following *mitāhāra,* we will be able to better feed everyone on the planet; fewer will be hungry. We won't have such extreme inequalities of excessive diet and inadequate diet, the incongruity of gluttony and malnutrition. We will have global moderation. The Hindu view is that we are part of ecology, an intricate part of the planet. Our physical body is a species here with rights equal to a flea, cockroach, bird, snake, a fish, a small animal or an elephant.

Diet and Good Health

By following *mitāhāra* you can be healthier, and you can be wealthier. A lot of money is wasted in the average family on food that could go toward many other things the family needs or wants. If you are healthier, you save on doctor bills, and because this also helps in *sādhana* and meditation, you will be healthy, happy and holy. Overeating repels one from spiritual *sādhana,* because the body becomes slothful and lazy, having to digest so much food and run it through its system. Eating is meant to nourish the body with vitamins and minerals to keep it functioning. It is not meant for mere personal, sensual pleasure. A slothful person naturally does not have the inclination to advance himself through education and meditation, and is unable to do anything but a simple, routine job.

We recently heard of a Western science lab study that fed two groups of rats different portions of food. Those who were allowed to have any amount of food they could eat lived a normal rat life span. Those who were given half that much lived twice as long. This so impressed the scientists that they immediately dropped their own calorie input and lost many pounds, realizing that a long, healthy life could be attained by not eating so much.

People on this planet are divided in two groups, as delineated by states of consciousness. The most obvious group is those ruled by lower consciousness, which proliferates deceit and dishonesty and the confusion in life that these bring, along with fear, anger, jealousy and the subsequent remorseful emotions that follow. On the purer side are those in higher consciousness, ruled by the powers of reason and memory, willpower, good judgment, universal love, compassion and more. A vegetarian diet helps to open the inner man to the outer person and brings forth higher consciousness. Eating meat, fish, fowl and eggs opens the doors to lower consciousness. It's as simple as that. A vegetarian diet creates the right chemistry for spiritual life. Other diets create a different chemistry, which affects your endocrine glands and your entire system all day long. A vegetarian diet helps your system all day long. Food is chemistry, and chemistry affects consciousness; and if our goal is higher consciousness, we have to provide the chemistry that evokes it.

Take Charge of Your Body

There is a wonderful breathing exercise you can perform to aid the digestion and elimination of food by stimulating the internal fire. Breathe in through your nose a normal breath, and out through your nose very fast while pulling the stomach in. Then relax your stomach and again breathe in naturally and then out quickly by pulling the stomach in to force the air out of the lungs. Do this for one minute, then rest for one minute, then do it again. Then rest for a minute and do it again. About three repetitions is generally enough to conquer indigestion or constipation. This *prāṇāyāma* amplifies the heat of the body and stimulates the fire that digests food and eliminates waste. It is especially good for those who are rather sedentary and do a lot of intellectual work, whose energies are in the intellect and may not be addressing their digestive needs adequately.

Take charge of your own body and see that it is working right, is healthy and you are eating right. If you do overindulge, then compensate by fasting occasionally and performing physical disciplines. Most people have certain cravings and desires which they permit themselves to indulge in, whether it be sweets or rich, exotic foods or overly spiced foods. Discovering and moderating such personal preferences and desires is part of the spiritual path. If you find you overindulge in jelly beans, cashew nuts, licorice, chocolate, varieties of soft drinks or exotic imported coffee, moderate those appetites. Then you are controlling the entire desire nature of the instinctive mind in the process. That is a central process of spiritual unfoldment—to control and moderate such desires.

The *ṛishis* of yore taught us to restrain desire. They used the words *restrain* and *moderate* rather than *suppress* or *eliminate*. We must remember that to restrain and moderate desire allows the energy which is restrained and moderated to enliven higher *chakras*, giving rise to creativity and intuition that will actually better mankind, one's own household and the surrounding community.

The *ṛishis* have given us great knowledge to help us know

what to do. Study your body and your diet and find out what works for you. Find out what foods give you indigestion and stop eating those things. But remember that eating right, in itself, is not spiritual life. In the early stages seekers often become obsessed with finding the perfect diet. That is a stage they have to go through in learning. They have to find out what is right for them. But it should balance out to a simple routine of eating to live, not living to eat.

Reasons for Vegetarianism

Vegetarianism has for thousands of years been a principle of health and environmental ethics throughout India. Though Muslim and Christian colonization radically undermined and eroded this ideal, it remains to this day a cardinal ethic of Hindu thought and practice. A subtle sense of guilt persists among Hindus who eat meat, and there exists an ongoing controversy on this issue. The Sanskrit for vegetarianism is *śākāhāra,* and one following a vegetarian diet is a *śākāhārī.* The term for meat-eating is *mānsāhāra,* and the meat-eater is called *mānsāhārī. Āhāra* means "food" or "diet," *śāka* means "vegetable," and *mānsa* means "meat" or "flesh."

Amazingly, I have heard people define *vegetarian* as a diet which excludes the meat of animals but does permit fish and eggs. But what really is vegetarianism? It is living only on foods produced by plants, with the addition of dairy products. Vegetarian foods include grains, fruits, vegetables, legumes, milk, yogurt, cheese and butter. The strictest vegetarians, known as vegans, exclude all dairy products. Natural, fresh foods, locally grown without insecticides or chemical fertilizers are preferred. A vegetarian diet does not include meat, fish, shellfish, fowl or eggs. For good health, even certain vegetarian foods are minimized: frozen and canned foods, highly processed foods, such as white rice, white sugar and white flour; and "junk" foods and beverages—those with abundant chemical additives, such as artificial sweeteners, colorings, flavorings and preservatives.

In the past fifty years millions of meat-eaters have made the decision to stop eating the flesh of other creatures. There are five major motivations for such a decision.

1) Many become vegetarian purely to uphold *dharma*, as the first duty to God and God's creation as defined by Vedic scripture.

2) Some abjure meat-eating because of the *karmic* consequences, knowing that by involving oneself, even indirectly, in the cycle of inflicting injury, pain and death by eating other creatures, one must in the future experience in equal measure the suffering caused.

3) Spiritual consciousness is another reason. Food is the source of the body's chemistry, and what we ingest affects our consciousness, emotions and experiential patterns. If one wants to live in higher consciousness, in peace and happiness and love for all creatures, then he cannot eat meat, fish, shellfish, fowl or eggs. By ingesting the grosser chemistries of animal foods, one introduces into the body and mind anger, jealousy, fear, anxiety, suspicion and a terrible fear of death, all of which are locked into the flesh of butchered creatures.

4) Medical studies prove that a vegetarian diet is easier to digest, provides a wider range of nutrients and imposes fewer burdens and impurities on the body. Vegetarians are less susceptible to all the major diseases that afflict contemporary humanity, and thus live longer, healthier, more productive lives. They have fewer physical complaints, less frequent visits to the doctor, fewer dental problems and smaller medical bills. Their immune system is stronger, their bodies purer and more refined, and their skin clearer, more supple and smooth.

5) Finally, there is the ecological reason. Planet Earth is suffering. In large measure, the escalating loss of species, destruction of ancient rainforests to create pasture lands

for livestock, loss of topsoil and the consequent increase of water impurities and air pollution have all been traced to the single fact of meat in the human diet. No single decision that we can make as individuals or as a race can have such a dramatic effect on the improvement of our planetary ecology as the decision to not eat meat. Many conscious of the need to save the planet for future generations have made this decision for this reason and this reason alone.

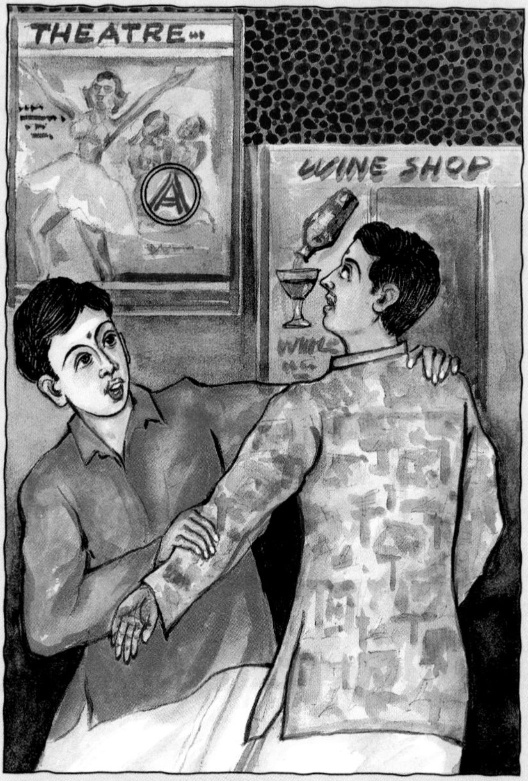

A man finds his friend outside an X-rated theater and urges him not to sink into a low-minded sensual life.

Summary of the Tenth Restraint

Uphold the ethic of purity, avoiding impurity in mind, body and speech. Maintain a clean, healthy body. Keep a pure, uncluttered home and workplace. Act virtuously. Keep good company, never mixing with adulterers, thieves or other impure people. Keep away from pornography and violence. Never use harsh, angered or indecent language. Worship devoutly. Meditate daily.

THE TENTH RESTRAINT

Purity

Śaucha शौच

PURITY, *ŚAUCHA,* NUMBER TEN OF THE *YAMAS,* IS THE OUTCOME OF RESTRAINING OURSELVES IN ALL THE OTHER NINE. PURITY IS THE NATURAL HERITAGE OF MEN AND WOMEN, disciplined in mind and body, who think before they speak, speaking only that which is true, kind, helpful and necessary. People whose thoughts are pure—and this means being in line with the *yamas* and *niyamas*—and whose bodies are free from incompatible alien obstructions, are naturally happy, content and ready to perform *japa. Japa yoga* lifts the spiritual energies and annihilates pride and arrogance by awakening within the superconscious areas of the mind an extraterrestrial intelligence, far surpassing the ordinary intellect one would encounter in the schools and universities of the present day. To be pure in mind means to have a bright, luminous aura filled with the pastel hues of the primary and secondary colors under every circumstance and life situation. Those who practice this restraint have realized that thoughts create and manifest into situations, actual physical happenings. Therefore, they are careful what they think and to whom they direct their thoughts.

A clean personal environment, wearing clean clothes, bathing often, keeping the room spotless where you meditate, breathing clean air, letting fresh air pass through your house, is all very important in the fulfillment of purity. *Śaucha* also includes partaking of clean food, which ideally is freshly picked food, cooked within minutes of the picking. There are creative forces, preservation forces and forces of dissolution. The preservation force is in the continued growing of a fruit or a leafy vegetable. It reaches its normal size and if not picked remains on the plant and is preserved by the life of that plant. As soon as it is picked, the force of dissolution, *mumia,* sets in. Therefore, the food should be cooked and eaten as soon after picking as possible, before the *mumia* force gets strong. *Mumia,* as it causes the breakdown of the cells, is an impure force. When we constantly eat food that is on the breakdown, the body is sluggish, the mind is sluggish and the tongue is loose, and we say things we don't mean. Many unhappy, depressed situations result from people eating a predominance of frozen foods, processed foods, canned foods, convenience foods, which are all in the process of *mumia.*

Clean clothing is very important. One feels invigorated and happy wearing clean clothing. Even hanging clothing out in the sunlight for five minutes a day cleanses and refreshes it. An incredible amount of body waste is eliminated through the skin and absorbed by the clothing we wear. It is commonly thought that clothing does not need to be cleaned unless it has been dirtied or soiled with mud, dirt or stains. Very little concern is given to the body odors and wastes that are exuded through the pores, then caught and held by the fabric. Small wonder it's so refreshing to put on clean clothing. The sun and fresh air can eliminate much of the body waste and freshen up any garment.

Keeping Pure Surroundings

Cleaning the house is an act of purifying one's immediate environment. Each piece of furniture, as well as the doorways and the walls, catches and holds the emanations of the human aura of each individual in the home, as well as each of its visitors. This residue must be wiped away through dusting and cleaning. This regular attentiveness keeps each room sparkling clean and actinic. Unless this is done, the rooms of the home become overpowering to the consciousness of the individuals who live within them as their auras pick up the old accumulated feelings of days gone by. Small wonder that a dirty room can depress you, and one freshly cleaned can invigorate.

In these years, when both mother and father work in the outside world, the house is often simply where they sleep and eat. But if a home receives all of the daily attentions of cleaning it sparkly bright, both astrally and physically, it becomes a welcoming place and not an empty shell. The *devas* can live within a home that is clean and well regulated, where the routine of breakfast, lunch and dinner is upheld, where early morning devotionals are performed and respected, a home which the family lives together within, eats together within, talks together within, worships together within. Such a home is the abode of the *devas.* Other kinds of homes are the abodes of *asuric* forces and disincarnate entities bound to Earth by lower desires.

It is very important that the *saṁskāras* are performed properly within a *śaucha* abode, particularly the *antyeshṭi,* or funeral, ceremonies so as to restore purity in the home after a death. Birth and death require the family to observe a moratorium of at least thirty-one days during which they do not enter the temple or the shrine room. Such obligatory ritual customs are important to follow for those wishing to restrain their desires and perfect *śaucha* in body, mind and speech, keeping good company, keeping the mind pure and avoiding impure thoughts.

Purity and impurity can be discerned in the human aura. We see purity in the brilliancy of the aura of one who is restraining and disciplining the lower instinctive nature, as outlined in these *yamas* and *niyamas.* His aura is bright with white rays from his soul lightening up the various hues and colors of his moods and emotions. Impure people have black shading in the colors of their aura as they go through their moods and emotions. Black in the aura is from the lower worlds, the worlds of darkness, of the *tala chakras* below the *mūlādhāra.*

Wholesome Company

It is unfortunate that at this time in the Kali Yuga there are more people on the Earth in important positions who have risen into physical birth from the Narakaloka, the world of darkness, than have descended from the Devaloka, the world of light. Therefore, they are strong as they band together in anger, corruption, deceit and contempt for the Devaloka people, who live in the *chakras* above the *mūlādhāra.* It is important for the Devaloka people to ferret out who is good company and who is not. They should not presume that they can effect any sustainable changes in the Narakaloka people. And they need to know that the *asuric* people, bound in anger, greed, jealousy, contempt, covetousness and lust, can make and sustain a difference within the *devonic* people, bringing them down into their world, torturing and tormenting them with their callous, cruel and insensitive feelings. To sustain *śaucha,* it is important to surround oneself with good, *devonic* company, to have the discrimination to know one type of person from another. Too many foolish, sensitive souls, thinking their spirituality could lift a soul from the world of darkness, have walked in where even the Mahādevas do not tread and the *devas* fear to tread, only to find themselves caught in that very world, through the deceit and conniving of the cleverly cunning. Let's not be foolish. Let's discriminate between higher consciousness and lower consciousness. Higher-consciousness people should surround themselves with higher-consciousness people to fulfill *śaucha.*

Changing to a purer life can be so simple. You don't have to give up anything. Just learn to like things that are better. That is the spirit of purity. When you give up something because you think you should give it up, that creates strain. Instead, search for a better life; search for *śaucha.* From *tamasic* eating we go to *rajasic* eating, and because *sattvic* food tastes better and makes us feel better, we also leave much of the *rajasic* food behind. Are not all persons on this planet driven by desire? Yes, indeed. Then let's redirect desire and let our desires perfect us. Let us learn to desire the more tasty, *sattvic* foods, the more sublime sounds, the most perfect things we can see, more than the gross, exciting and reprehensible, the desires for which will fade away when we attach ourselves to something better. Let our desires perfect us. The ultra-democratic dream of life, liberty and the pursuit of happiness we can use as a New-Age goal and pursue the happiness of something better than what we are doing now that is bad for us. Let's go forward with the spirit of moving onward.

A devotee told me, "I gave up coffee because coffee is a stimulant and a depressant. I stopped eating meat because meat is a cholesterol-creating killer and forest decimator." Another approach would be to give up coffee because you have found a beverage that is better. Test all beverages. Some have found that coffee gives you indigestion and green tea helps you digest your food, especially oily foods and foods that remain in your stomach undigested through the night. It also tastes good. Others have found that freshly picked, nutritious vegetables, especially when cooked within minutes of the picking, give more life and energy than eating dead meat that has been refrigerated or preserved. Still others have found that if you kill an animal and eat it fresh, it has more nutritive value than killing it, refrigerating it, preserving it, then cooking it to death again!

Be mature about it when you give something up. The immature spiritual person will want everyone else to give it up, too. The spiritually mature person quietly surrenders it because it is simply his personal choice and then goes on with his life. The spiritually immature person will make a big issue of giving anything up and want everyone to know about it.

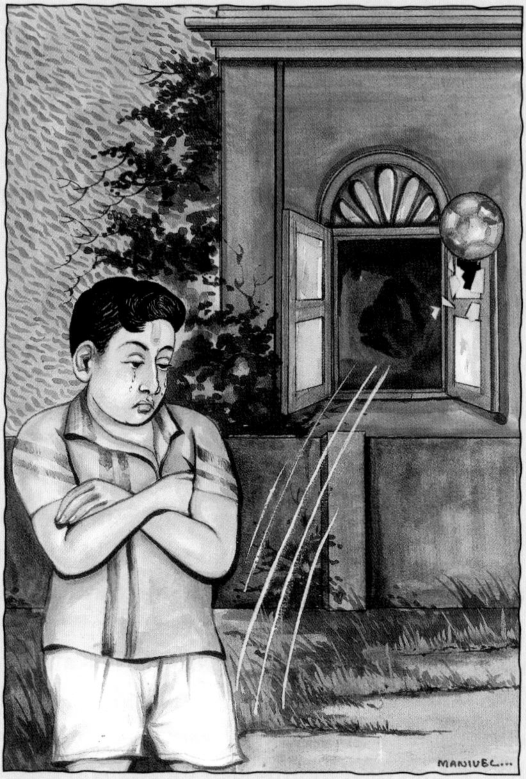

The boy's tears show his remorse, hrī, *at having accidentally broken a neighbor's window.*

❀

Summary of the First Observance

Allow yourself the expression of remorse, being modest and showing shame for misdeeds. Recognize your errors, confess and make amends. Sincerely apologize to those hurt by your words or deeds. Resolve all contention before sleep. Seek out and correct your faults and bad habits. Welcome correction as a means to bettering yourself. Do not boast. Shun pride and pretension.

THE FIRST OBSERVANCE

Remorse & Modesty

Hrī ह्री

H*RĪ*, THE FIRST OF THE TEN *NIYAMAS,* OR PRACTICES, IS REMORSE: BEING MODEST AND SHOWING SHAME FOR MISDEEDS, SEEKING THE *GURU'S* GRACE TO BE RELEASED FROM sorrows through the understanding that he gives, based on the ancient *sampradāya,* doctrinal lineage, he preaches. Remorse could be the most misunderstood and difficult to practice of all of the *niyamas,* because we don't have very many role models today for modesty or remorse. In fact, the role for imitation in today's world is just the opposite. This is reflected in television, on film, in novels, magazines, newspapers and all other kinds of media. In today's world, brash, presumptuous, prideful—that's how one must be. That's the role model we see everywhere. In today's world, arrogant—that's how one must be. That's the role model we see everywhere. Therefore, to be remorseful or even to show modesty would be a sign of weakness to one's peers, family and friends.

Modesty is portrayed in the media as a trait of people that are gauche, inhibited, undeveloped emotionally or not well educated. And remorse is portrayed in the world media as a characteristic of one who "doesn't have his act together," is unable to rationalize away wrongdoings, or who is not clever enough to find a scapegoat to pin the blame on. Though modesty and remorse are the natural qualities of the soul, when the soul does exhibit these qualities, there is a natural tendency to suppress them.

But let's look on the brighter side. There is an old saying, "Some people teach us what to do, and other people teach us what not to do." The modern media, at least most of it, is teaching us what not to do. Its behavior is based on other kinds of philosophy—secular humanism, materialism, existentialism, crime and punishment, terrorism—in its effort to report and record the stories of the day. Sometimes we can learn quite a lot by seeing the opposite of what we want to learn. The proud and arrogant people portrayed on TV nearly always have their fall. This is always portrayed extremely well and is very entertaining. In their heart of hearts, people really do not admire the prideful person or his display of arrogance, so they take joy in seeing him get his just due. People, in their heart of hearts, do admire the modest person, the truthful person, the patient person, the steadfast person, the compassionate person who shows contentment and the fullness of well-being on his face and in his behavioral patterns.

We Hindus who understand these things know that *hrī*, remorse, is to be practiced at every opportunity. One of the most acceptable ways to practice *hrī*, even in today's society, is to say in a heartfelt way, "I'm sorry." Everyone will accept this. Even the most despicable, prideful, arrogant, self-centered person will melt just a little under the two magic words "I'm sorry." When apologizing, explain to the person you hurt or wronged how you have realized that there was a better way and ask for his forgiveness. If the person is too proud or arrogant to forgive, you have done your part and can go your way. The burden of the quandary you have put him into now lies solely with him. He will think about it, justify how and why and what he should not forgive until the offense melts from his mind and his heart softens. It takes as much time for a hardened heart to soften as it does for a piece of ice to melt in a refrigerator. Even when it does, his pride may never let him give you the satisfaction of knowing he has forgiven you. But you can tell. Watch for softening in the eyes when you meet, a less rigid mouth and the tendency to suppress a wholesome smile.

Body Language and Conscience

There is another way to show remorse for misdeeds. That is by performing *seva,* religious service, for persons you have wronged. Give them gifts, cook them food. Some people are unreachable by words, too remote for an apology, which might even lead to an argument, and then the wrong would perpetuate itself. Be extra polite to such people. Hold the door open as they walk through. Never miss an opportunity to be kind and serve. Say kind words about them behind their back. The praise must be true and timely. Mere flattery would be unacceptable. This kind of silent behavior shows repentance, shows remorse, shows that you have reconsidered your actions and found that they need improvement, and the improvement is shown by your actions now and into the future.

Often people think that showing shame and modesty and remorse for misdeeds is simply hanging your head. Well, really, anyone can do this, but it's not genuine if the head is not pulled down by the tightening of the strings of the heart, if shame is not felt so deeply that one cannot look another in the eye. When the hanging of the head is genuine, everyone will know it and seek to lift you up out of the predicament. But just to hang your head for a while and think you're going to get away with it in today's world, no. In today's world, people are a little too perceptive, and will not admire you, as they will suspect pretense.

There is an analogy in the Śaivite tradition that compares the unfolding soul to wheat. When young and growing, the stalks of wheat stand tall and proud, but when mature their heads bend low under the weight of the grains they yield. Similarly, man is self-assertive, arrogant and vain only in the early stages of his spiritual growth. As he matures and yields the harvest of divine knowledge, he too bends his head. Body language has to truly be the language of the body. It's a dead giveaway. Body language is the language of the mind being expressed through the body. Let there be no doubt about this. To cry, expressing remorse—the crying should not be forced. Many people can cry on cue. We must not think that the soul of the observer is not perceptive enough to know the difference between real tears and a glandular disturbance causing watering of the eyes.

Hrī is regret that one has done things against the *dharma*, or against conscience. There are three kinds of conscience—one built on right knowledge, one built on semi-right knowledge and one built on wrong knowledge. The soul has to work through these three gridworks within the subconscious mind to give its message. Those who have been raised with the idea that an injustice should be settled by giving back another injustice might actually feel a little guilty when they fail to do this. Those who are in a quandary of what to do, what is right and what is wrong, remain in confusion because they have only semi-right knowledge in their subconscious mind.

We cannot confuse guilt and its messages with the message that comes from the soul. Guilt is the message of the instinctive mind, the *chakras* below the *mūlādhāra*. Many people who live in the lower worlds of darkness feel guilty and satisfy that guilt through retaliation. This is the eye for an eye-for-an-eye, tooth-for-a-tooth approach. This is not right conscience; it is not the soul speaking. This is not higher consciousness, and it is certainly not the inner being of light looking out of the windows of the *chakras* above the *mūlādhāra*. Why, even domesticated animals feel guilty. It is a quality of the instinctive mind.

True conscience is of the soul, an impulse rushing through a mind that has been impregnated with right knowledge, *Vedic, Āgamic* knowledge, or the knowledge that is found in these *yamas* and *niyamas*, restraints and practices. When the true knowledge of *karma* is understood, reincarnation, *saṁsāra* and *Vedic dharma*, then true remorse is felt, which is a corrective mechanism of the soul. This remorse immediately imprints upon the lower mind the right knowledge of the *dharma*—how, where and why the person has strayed and the methodology of getting quickly and happily back to the path and proceeding onward. There is no guilt felt here, but there is a sense of spiritual responsibility, and a driving urge to bring *dharma,* the sense of spiritual duty, more fully into one's life, thus filling up the lack that the misdeeds manifested through adhering to these twenty restraints and practices and the *Vedic* path of *dharma,* which is already known within the bedrock of right knowledge, firmly planted within the inner mind of the individual.

Compensating for Misdeeds

The soul's response to wrong action comes of its own force, unbidden, when the person is a free soul, not bound by many materialistic duties—even while doing selfless service—which can temporarily veil and hold back the spontaneous actions of the soul if done for the expectant praise that may follow. The held-back, spontaneous action of the soul would, therefore, burst forth during personal times of *sādhana,* meditation or temple worship. The bursting forth would be totally unbidden, and resolutions would follow in the wake. For those immersed in heavy *prārabdha karma*s, going through a period of their life cycle when difficult *karmic* patterns are manifesting, it will be found that the soul's spontaneity is triple-veiled even though the subconscious mind is impregnated with right knowledge. To gain absolution and release, to gain peace of mind, one should perform pilgrimage, spiritual retreat, the practice of *mauna,* recitation of *mantras* through *japa,* deep meditation and, best of all, the *vāsanā daha tantra.* These practices will temporarily pierce the veils of *māyā* and let the light shine in, bringing understanding, solutions and direction for future behavior.

Having hurt another through wrongdoing, one has to pay back in proportion to the injury, not a rupee less and not a rupee more. The moment the healing is complete, the scar will mysteriously vanish. This is the law. It is a mystical law. And while there are any remaining scars, which are memories impregnated with emotion, much work has to be done. Each one must find a way to be nice if he has been not nice, say kind words if previous words have been unkind, issue forth good feelings if the feelings previously exuded were nasty, inharmonious and unacceptable. Just as a responsible doctor or nurse must bring the healing to culmination, so the wrongdoer must deal with his wrongdoing, his crime against *dharma*, his crime against right knowledge, Vedic-Āgamic precepts, his crime against the *yamas* and *niyamas*, restraints and practices, which are in themselves right knowledge—a digest of the *Vedas*, we might say. He must deal with his wrongdoings, his errors, within himself until rightness, *santosha*, returns.

There are no magic formulas. Each one must find his own way to heal himself and others until the troublesome situation disappears from his own memory. This is why the practice called *vāsanā daha tantra*, writing down memories and burning them in a fire to release the emotion from the deep subconscious, has proven to be a solution uncomparable to any other. Only in this way will he know that, by whatever method he has applied, he has healed the one he wronged. True forgiveness is the greatest eraser, the greatest harmonizer. It is this process of misdeeds against *dharma*, followed by shame and remorse, as people interrelate with one another, that moves them forward in their evolution toward their ultimate goal of *mukti*.

The Japanese, unlike most of the rest of the world, have a great sense of loss of face, and a Japanese businessman will resign if he has shamed his family or his country. This is *hrī* and is very much ingrained in the Japanese society, which is based on Buddhist precepts. Buddhism itself is the outgrowth into the family community from a vast monastic order; whereas Hinduism is a conglomerate of many smaller religions, some of which are not outgrowths of a monastic community. Therefore, *hrī* is an integral part of the culture of Japan. They have maintained this and other cultural precepts, as the Buddhist monastic orders are still influential throughout Asia.

A materialist who loses face smiles and simply puts on another mask and continues as if nothing had ever happened. The saying goes, "Change your image and get on with life." No shame, repentance or reconciliation is shown by such people, as is so often portrayed on American television, and much worse, as it actually happens all the time in public life.

Humility, Shame and Shyness

The Hindu monastic has special disciplines in regard to remorse. If he doesn't, he is an impostor. If he is seen struggling to observe it and unable to accomplish it all the time, he is still a good monastic. If he shows no remorse, modesty or shame for misdeeds for long periods of time, even though he continues apparently in the performance of no misdeeds, the abbot of the monastery would know that he is suppressing many things, living a personal life, avoiding confrontation and obscuring that which is obvious to himself with a smile and the words, "Yes, everything is all right with me. The meditations are going fine. I get along beautifully with all of my brothers." You would know that this is a "mission impossible," and that it is time to effect certain tests to break up the nest of the enjoyable routine and of keeping out of everybody's way, of not participating creatively in the entire community, but just doing one's job and keeping out of trouble. The test would bring him out in the open, into counseling sessions, so that he himself would see that his clever pride had led him to a spiritual standstill. A monastery is no place to settle down and live. It is a place to be on one's toes and advance. One must always live as if on the eve of one's departure.

Another side of *hrī* is being bashful, shy, unpretentious. The undeveloped person and the fully developed, wise person may develop the same qualities of being bashful, shy, unpretentious, cautious. In the former, these qualities are the products of ignorance produced by underexposure, and in the latter, they are the products of the wisdom or cleverness produced by overexposure. Genuine modesty and unpretentiousness are not what actors on the stage would portray, they are qualities that one cannot act out, qualities of the soul.

Shyness used to be thought of as a feminine quality, but not anymore, since the equality of men and women has been announced as the way that men and women should be. Both genders should be aggressive, forceful, to meet and deal with situations on equal terms. This is seen today in the West, in the East, in the North and the South. This is a façade which covers the soul, producing stress in both men and women. A basically shy man or woman, feeling he or she has to be aggressive, works his or her way into a stressful condition. I long ago found that stress in itself is a byproduct of not being secure in what one is doing. But this is the world today, at this time in the Kali Yuga. If everything that is happening were reasonable and could be easily understood, it certainly wouldn't be the Kali Yuga.

If people are taught and believe that their spiritual pursuits are foremost, then, yes, they should be actively aggressive—but as actively passive and modest as well, because of their spiritual pursuits. Obviously, if they are performing *sādhanas*, they will intuitively know the proper timing for each action. Remorse, or modesty, certainly does not mean one must divorce oneself from the ability to move the forces of the external world, or be a wimpy kind of impotent person. It does mean that there is a way of being remorseful, showing shame, being humble, of resolving situations when they do go wrong so that you can truly "get on with life" and not be bound by emotionally saturated memories of the past. Those who are bound by the past constantly remember the past and relive the emotions connected with it. Those who are free from the past remember the future and move the forces of all three worlds for a better life for themselves and for all mankind. This is the potent Vedic *hrī*. This is true remorse, humility and modesty. This is *hrī*, which is not a weakness but a spiritual strength. And all this is made practical and permanent by subconscious journaling, *vāsanā daha tantra*, which releases creative energy and does not inhibit it.

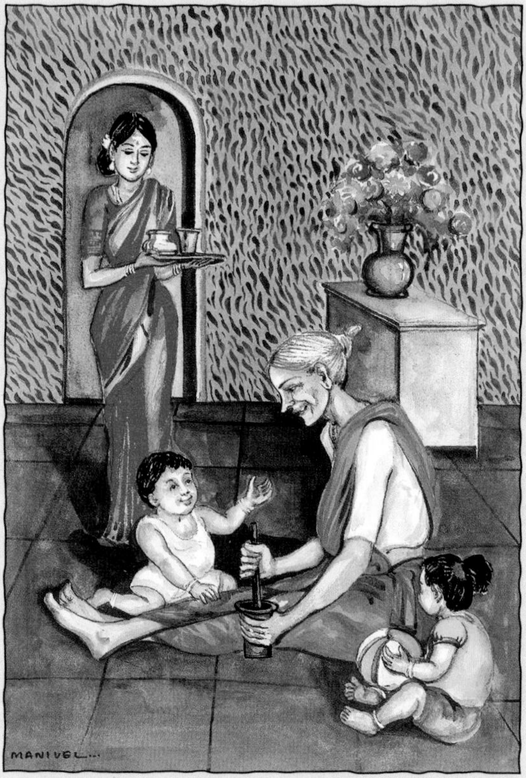

Three generations living at home, enjoying one another, happy, fulfilled and content in their simple life.

❁

Summary of the Second Observance

Nurture contentment, seeking joy and serenity in life. Be happy, smile and uplift others. Live in constant gratitude for your health, your friends and your belongings. Don't complain about what you don't possess. Identify with the eternal You, rather than mind, body or emotions. Keep the mountaintop view that life is an opportunity for spiritual progress. Live in the eternal now.

THE SECOND OBSERVANCE

Contentment

Santosha सन्तोष

CONTENTMENT, *SANTOSHA,* IS THE SECOND *NIYAMA*. HOW DO WE PRACTICE CONTENTMENT? SIMPLY DO NOT HARM OTHERS BY THOUGHT, WORD OR DEED. AS A PRACTItioner of *ahiṁsā,* noninjury, you can sleep contentedly at night and experience *santosha* then and through the day. Contentment is a quality that everyone wants, and buys things to obtain—"Oh, if I only had my house redecorated, I would be content." "A new wardrobe would content me, give me joy and serenity." "To be content, I must have a vacation and get away from it all. There I can live the serene life and have joyous experiences."

The *dharmic* way is to look within and bring out the latent contentment that is already there by doing nothing to inhibit its natural expression, as *santosha,* the mood of the soul, permeates out through every cell of the physical body. Contentment is one of the most difficult qualities to obtain, and is well summed up within our food blessing *mantra,* from the *Śukla Yajur Veda, Īsa Upanishad* invocation, "That is fullness. Creation is fullness. From that fullness flows this world's fullness. This fullness issues from that fullness, yet that fullness remains full." This joy we seek is the joy of fullness, lacking nothing.

Life is meant to be lived joyously. There is in much of the world the belief that life is a burden, a feeling of penitence, that it is good to suffer, good for the soul. In fact, spiritual life is not that way at all. The existentialist would have you believe that depression, rage, fear and anguish are the foremost qualities of the human temper and expression. The communists used to have us believe that joy and serenity as the outgrowth of religion are just an opiate of the people, a narcotic of unreality. The Semitic religions of the Near East would have us believe that suffering is good for the soul, and there is not much you can do about it. The Śaivite Hindu perspective is that contentment is a reflection of centeredness, and discontentment is a reflection of externalized consciousness and ramified desire.

Maintaining joy and serenity in life means being content with your surroundings, be they meager or lavish. Be content with your money, be it a small amount or a large amount. Be content with your health. Bear up under ailments and be thankful that they are not worse than they are. Protect your health if it is good. It is a valuable treasure. Be content with your friends. Be loyal to those who are your long-time, trusted companions. Basically, contentment, *santosha,* is freedom from desire gained by redirecting the forces of desire and making a beautiful life within what one already has in life.

The rich seeking more riches are not content. The famous seeking more fame are not content. The learned seeking more knowledge are not content. Being content with what you have does not mean you cannot discriminate and seek to progress in life. It doesn't mean you should not use your willpower and fulfill your plans.

It does mean you should not become upset while you are striving toward your goals, frustrated or unhappy if you do not get what you want. The best striving is to keep pushing along the natural unfoldment of positive trends and events in your life, your family life and your business. Contentment is working within your means with what is available to you, living within your income, being grateful for what you have, and not unhappy over what you lack.

There are many frustrated souls on the path who torment themselves no end and walk around with long faces because they estimate they are not unfolding spiritually fast enough. They have set goals of Self Realization for themselves far beyond their abilities to immediately obtain. If people say, "I am not going to do anything that will not make me peaceful or that will threaten my peace of mind," how will they get anywhere? That is not the idea of *santosha.* True *santosha* is seeing all-pervasiveness of the one divine power everywhere. The light within the eyes of each person is that divine power. With this in mind, you can go anywhere and do anything. Contentment is there, inside you, and needs to be brought out. It is a spiritual power. So, yes, do what makes you content. But know that contentment really transcends worrying about the challenges that face you. *Santosha* is being peaceful in any situation. The stronger you are in *santosha,* the greater the challenges you can face and still remain quiet on the inside, peaceful and content, poised like a hummingbird hovering over a flower.

Keeping Peace in the Home

Santosha is the goal; *dharma,* good conduct, remains the director of how you should act and respond to fulfill your *karma.* This goal is attainable by following the ten Vedic restraints: not harming others by thought, word or deed, refraining from lying, not entering into debt, being tolerant with people and circumstance, overcoming changeableness and indecision, not being callous, cruel or insensitive to other people's feelings. Above all, never practice deception. Don't eat too much. Maintain a vegetarian diet for purity and clarity of mind. Watch carefully what you think and how you express it through words. All of these restraints must be captured and practiced within the lifestyle before the natural contentment, the *santosha,* the pure, serene nature, of the soul can shine forth. Therefore, the practice to attain *santosha* is to fulfill the *yamas.* Proceed with confidence; failure is an impossibility.

I was asked by a cyberspace cadet among our Internet congregation, "Where do we let off steam? Mom works, dad works, the kids are in school, and when everyone comes home, everyone lets off a little steam, and everyone understands." My answer is don't let off steam in the home. The home is a sanctuary of the entire family. It should have an even higher standard of propriety than the office, the factory or the corporate workplace. When we start being too casual at home and letting off steam, we say things that perhaps we shouldn't. We may think the rest of the family understands, but they don't. Feelings get hurt. We break up the vibration of the home. Young people also let off steam in school, thus inhibiting their own education. They behave in a way in the classroom that they would not in a corporate office, and who is hurt but themselves? It's amazing how quickly people shape up their behavior when they sign a contract, when they get a job in a corporate office. They read the manual, they obey it and they are nice to everyone. This is the way it should be within the home. The home should be maintained at a higher standard than the corporate office.

The wonderful thing about Hinduism is that we don't let off steam at home; we let our emotions pour out within the Hindu temple. The Hindu temple is the place where we can relate to the Gods and the Goddesses and express ourselves within ourselves. It's just between ourselves and the Deity. In a Hindu temple there may be, all at the same time, a woman worshiper crying in a corner, not far away a young couple laughing among themselves with their children, and nearby someone else arguing with the Gods. The Hindu temple allows the individual to let off steam but it is a controlled situation, controlled by the *pūjās,* the ceremony, the priesthood.

So as to not make more *karma* in this life by saying things we don't mean, having inflections in our voice that are hurtful to others, we must control the home, control ourselves in the workplace, keep the home at a higher vibration of culture and protocol than the workplace, and include the temple in our lives as a place to release our emotions and regain our composure.

It is making a lot of really bad *karma* that will come back in its stronger reaction later on in life for someone, the husband or wife or teenager, to upset the vibration of the home because of stress at school or in the workplace. It is counterproductive to work all day in a nice office, control the emotions and be productive, and then go home and upset the vibration within the home. After all, why is someone working? It's to create the home. Why is someone going to school? It's to eventually create a home. It is counterproductive to destroy that which one works all day to create. That's why I advise the professional mother, the professional father, the professional son and the professional daughter to use in the home the same good manners that are learned in the workplace, and build the vibration of the home even stronger than the vibration of the workplace, so that there is something inviting to come home to.

We have seen so many times, professionals, men and women, behave exquisitely in the workplace, but not so exquisitely at home, upset the home vibration, eventually destroying the home, breaking up the home. And we have seen, through the years, a very unhappy person in retirement, a very bitter person in retirement. No one wants him around, no one wants to have him in their home. Therefore, he winds up in some nursing home, and he dies forgotten.

The Sanātana Dharma and Śaiva Samayam must be alive in the home, must be alive in the office, must be alive in the temple, for us to have a full life. Where, then, do we vent our emotions, where do we let off steam, if not in our own home? The answer is, within the temple.

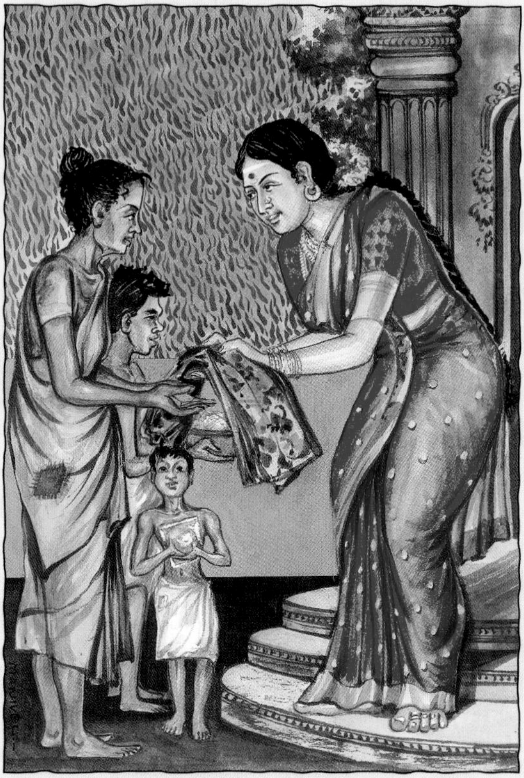

A well-to-do woman takes joy in giving food and clothing to needy neighbors in a selfless act of dāna.

Summary of the Third Observance

Be generous to a fault, giving liberally without thought of reward. Tithe, offering one-tenth of your gross income *(daśamāṁśa)* as God's money, to temples, *ashrams* and spiritual organizations. Approach the temple with offerings. Visit *gurus* with gifts in hand. Donate religious literature. Feed and give to those in need. Bestow your time and talents without seeking praise. Treat guests as God.

THE THIRD OBSERVANCE

Giving

Dāna दान

GIVING, *DĀNA*, IS THE THIRD GREAT RELIGIOUS PRACTICE, OR *NIYAMA*. IT IS IMPORTANT TO REMEMBER THAT GIVING FREELY OF ONE'S GOODS IN FULFILLING NEEDS, MAKING SOMEone happy or putting a smile on his face, mitigates selfishness, greed, avarice and hoarding. But the most important factor is "without thought of reward." The reward of joy and the fullness you feel is immediate as the gift passes from your two hands into the outstretched hands of the receiver. *Dāna* is often translated as "charity." But charity in modern context is a special kind of giving by those who have to those who have not. This is not the true spirit of *dāna*. The word *fulfillment* might describe *dāna* better. The fulfillment of giving that wells up within the giver as the gift is being prepared and as the gift is being presented and released, the fulfillment of the expectancy of the receiver or the surprise of the receiver, and the fullness that exists afterwards are all a part of *dāna*.

Daśamāṁśa, tithing, too, is a worthy form of *dāna*—giving God's money to a religious institution to fulfill with it God's work. One who is really fulfilling *dāna* gives *daśamāṁśa*, never goes to visit a friend or relative with empty hands, gives freely to relatives, children, friends, neighbors and business associates, all without thought of reward. The devotee who practices *dāna* knows fully that "you cannot give anything away." The law of *karma* will return it to you full measure at an appropriate and most needed time. The freer the gift is given, the faster it will return.

What is the proportionate giving after *daśamāṁśa*, ten

percent, has been deducted. It would be another two to five percent of one's gross income, which would be equally divided between cash and kind if someone wanted to discipline his *dāna* to that extent. That would be fifteen percent, approximately one sixth, which is the *makimai* established in South India by the Chettiar community around the Palani Temple and now practiced by the Malaka Chettiars of Malaysia.

If one were to take a hard look at the true spirit of *dāna* in today's society, the rich giving to religious institutions for a tax deduction are certainly giving with a thought of reward. Therefore, giving after the tax deductions are received and with no material benefits or rewards of any kind other than the fulfillment of giving is considered by the wise to be a true expression of *dāna.* Making something with one's own hands, giving in kind, is also a true expression of *dāna.* Giving a gift begrudgingly in return for another gift is, of course, mere barter. Many families barter their way through life in this way, thinking they are giving. But such gifts are cold, the fulfillment is empty, and the law of *karma* pays discounted returns.

Hospitality and Fullness

Hospitality is a vital part of fulfilling *dāna.* When guests come, they must be given hospitality, at least a mat to sit on and a glass of water to drink. These are obligatory gifts. You must never leave your guest standing, and you must never leave your guest thirsty. If a guest were to smell even one whiff from the kitchen of the scented curries of a meal being prepared, he must be asked four times to stay for the meal. He will politely refuse three times and accept on the fourth invitation. This is also an obligatory giving, for the guest is treated as God. God *Śiva's* veiling grace hides Śiva as He dresses in many costumes. He is a dancer, you know, and dancers wear many costumes. He will come as a guest to your home, unrecognizable. You might think it is your dear friend from a far-off place. That, too, is Śiva in another costume, and you must treat that guest as Śiva. Giving to Śiva Śiva's own creation in your mind brings the highest rewards through the law of *karma.*

Even if you think you are giving creatively, generously, looking for no rewards, but you are giving for a purpose, that *karma* will still pay you back with full interest and dividends. This is a positive use of the law of *karma.* It pays higher interest than any bank. This is not a selfish form of giving. It is the giving of the wise, because you know the law of *karma,* because you know the Sanātana Dharma—the divine, eternal laws. If you see a need that you can fill and have the impulse to give but recoil from giving, later, when you are in need, there will be someone who has the impulse to give to you but will recoil from giving. The wheels of *karma* grind slowly but exceedingly well the grains of actions, be they in thought, emotion or those of a physical nature. So, one can be quite selfish and greedy about wanting to practice *dāna* to accumulate the *puṇya* for the balance of this life, the life in-between lives, in the astral world, and for a good birth in the next incarnation. The practice of *dāna* is an investment in a better life, an investment that pays great dividends.

We are not limited by our poverty or wealth in practicing giving. No matter how poor you are, you can still practice it. You can give according to your means, your inspiration, your ability. When the fullness has reached its peak within you while preparing the gift, be it arranging a bouquet of freshly picked flowers, a tray of fruit, counting out coins, sorting a pile of bills or putting zeros on a check that you're writing, then you know that the gift is within your means. Gifts within your means and from your heart are the proper gifts.

The Selfish and Miserly

The virtue of *dāna* deals with the pragmatic physical transference of cash or kind. It is the foundation and the life blood of any other form of religious giving, such as giving of one's time. Many people rationalize, "I'll give my time to the temple. I'll wash the pots, scrub the floor and tidy up. But I can't afford to give of my limited wealth proportionate to what would be total fulfillment of giving." Basically, they have nothing better to do with their time, and to ease their own conscience, they volunteer a little work. There is no merit, no *puṇya*, in this, only demerit, *pāpa*. No, it's just the other way around. One who has perfected *dāna* in cash and in kind and is satisfied within this practice, this *niyama*, will then be able and willing to give of his time, to tithe ten percent of his time, and then give time over and above that to religious and other worthy causes. Shall we say that the perfection of *dāna* precedes *seva,* service?

What can be said of someone who is all wrapped up in his personal self: concealing his personal ego with a pleasant smile, gentle deeds, soft words, but who just takes care of "number one"? For instance, if living with ten people, he will cook for himself and not cook for the others. He gets situations confused, entertains mental arguments within himself and is always worried about the progress in his religious life. We would say he is still trying to work on the restraints—compassion, patience, sexual purity, moderate appetite—and has not yet arrived at number three on the chart of the practices called *niyamas.* Modern psychology would categorize him as self-centered, selfish, egotistical. To overcome this selfishness, assuming he gets the restraints in order, doing things for others would be the practice, seeing that everyone is fed first before he eats, helping out in every way he can, performing anonymous acts of kindness at every opportunity.

In an orthodox Hindu home, the traditional wife will follow the practice of arising in the morning before her husband, preparing his hot meal, serving him and eating only after he is finished; preparing his lunch, serving him and eating after he is finished; preparing his dinner, serving him and eating after he is finished, even if he returns home late. Giving to her husband is her fulfillment, three times a day. This is built into Hindu society, into Śaivite culture.

Wives should be allowed by their husbands to perform giving outside the home, too, but many are not. All too often, they are held down, embarrassed and treated almost like domestic slaves—given no money, given no things to give, disallowed to practice *dāna,* to tithe and give creatively without thought of reward. Such domineering, miserly and ignorant males will get their just due in the courts of *karma* at the moment of death and shortly after. The divine law is that the wife's *śakti* power, once released, makes her husband magnetic and successful in his worldly affairs, and their wealth accumulates. He knows from tradition that to release this *śakti* he must always fulfill all of the needs of his beloved wife and give her generously everything she wants.

Many Ways of Giving

There are so many ways of giving. Arising before the Sun comes up, greeting and giving *namaskāra* to the Sun is a part of Śaivite culture. *Dāna* is built into all aspects of Hindu life—giving to the holy man, giving to the astrologer, giving to the teacher, giving *dakshiṇā* to a *swāmī* or a *satguru* for his support, over and above all giving to his institution, over and above *daśamāṁśa,* over and above giving to the temple. If the *satguru* has satisfied you with the fullness of his presence, you must satisfy yourself in equal fullness in giving back. You can be happily fat as these two fullnesses merge within you. By giving to the *satguru,* you give him the satisfaction of giving to another, for he has no needs except the need to practice *dāna.*

Great souls have always taught that, among all the forms of giving, imparting the spiritual teachings is the highest. You can give money or food and provide for the physical aspects of the being, but if you can find a way to give the *dharma,* the illumined wisdom of the traditions of the Sanātana Dharma, then you are giving to the spirit of the person, to the soul. Many Hindus buy religious literature to give away, because *jñāna dāna,* giving wisdom, is the highest giving. Several groups in Malaysia and Mauritius gave away over 70,000 pieces of literature in a twenty-month period. Another group in the United States gave away 300,000 pieces of literature in the same period. Many pieces of that literature changed the lives of individuals and brought them into a great fullness of soul satisfaction. An electric-shock blessing would go out from them at the peak of their fulfillment and fill the hearts of all the givers. Giving through education is a glorious fulfillment for the giver, as well as for the receiver.

Wealthy men in India will feed twenty thousand people in the hopes that one enlightened soul who was truly hungry at that time might partake of this *dāna* and the *śakti* that arises within him at the peak-of his satisfaction will prepare for the giver a better birth in his next life. This is the great spirit of *anna yajñā,* feeding the masses.

Along with the gift comes a portion of the *karma* of the giver. There was an astrologer who when given more than his due for a *jyotisha* consultation would always give the excess to a nearby temple, as he did not want to assume any additional *karma* by receiving more than the worth of his predictions. Another wise person said, "I don't do the *antyeshṭi saṁskāra,* funeral rites, because I can't receive the *dāna* coming from that source of sadness. It would affect my family." Giving is also a way of balancing *karma,* of expressing gratitude for blessings received. A devotee explained, "I cannot leave the temple without giving to the *huṇḍi,* offering box, according to the fullness I have received as fullness from the temple." A gourmet once said, "I cannot leave the restaurant until I give gratuity to the waiter equaling the satisfaction I felt from the service he gave." This is *dāna*, this is giving, in a different form.

Children should be taught giving at a very young age. They don't yet have the ten restraints, the *yamas*, to worry about. They have not been corrupted by the impact of their own *prārabdha karmas*. Little children, even babies, can be taught *dāna*—giving to the temple, to holy ones, to one another, to their parents. They can be taught worship, recitation and, of course, contentment—told how beautiful they are when they are quiet and experiencing the joy of serenity. Institutions should also give, according to their means, to other institutions.

How Monks Fulfill *Dāna*

It is very important for *sādhus, sannyāsins, swāmīs, sādhakas*, any mendicant under vows, to perform *dāna*. True, they are giving all of their time, but that is fulfillment of their *vrata*. True, they are not giving *daśamāṁśa*, because they are not employed and have no income. For them, *dāna* is giving the unexpected in unexpected ways—serving tea for seven days to the tyrannical *sādhu* that assisted them by causing an attack of *āṇava*, of personal ego, within them, in thanks to him for being the channel of their *prārabdha karmas* and helping them in the next step of their spiritual unfoldment. *Dāna* is making an unexpected wreath of sacred leaves and flowers for one's *guru* and giving it at an unexpected time. *Dāna* is cooking for the entire group and not just for a few or for oneself alone.

When one has reached an advanced stage on the spiritual path, in order to go further, the law requires giving back what one has been given. Hearing oneself speak the divine teachings and being uplifted and fulfilled by filling up and uplifting others allows the budding adept to go through the next portal. Those who have no desire to counsel others, teach or pass on what they have learned are still in the learning stages themselves, traumatically dealing with one or more of the restraints and practices. The passing on of *jñāna,* wisdom, through counseling, consoling, teaching Sanātana Dharma and the only one final conclusion, monistic Śaiva Siddhānta, Advaita Īśvaravāda, is a fulfillment and completion of the cycle of learning for every monastic. This does not mean that he mouths indiscriminately what he has been told and memorized, but rather that he uses his philosophical knowledge in a timely way according the immediate needs of the listener, for wisdom is the timely application of knowledge.

The *dāna sādhana,* of course, for *sādhakas, sādhus, yogīs* and *swāmīs,* as they have no cash, is to practice *dāna* in kind, physical doing, until they are finally able to release the Sanātana Dharma from their own lips, as a natural outgrowth of their spirituality, spirit, *śakti,* bolt-of-lightening outpouring, because they are so filled up. Those who are filled up with the divine truths, in whom when that fullness is pressed down, compacted, locked in, it still oozes out and runs over, are those who pass on the Sanātana Dharma. They are the catalysts not only of this adult generation, but the one before it still living, and of children and the generations yet to come.

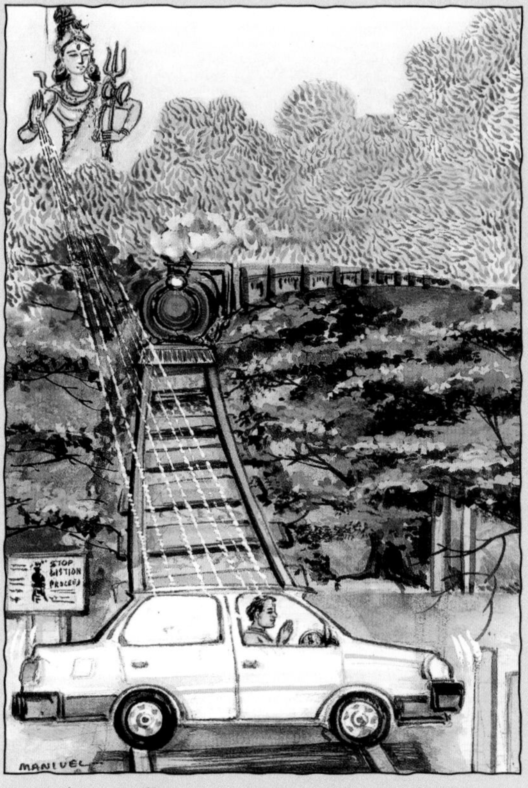

A man's car stalls as a train approaches. He holds to his faith, and Śiva, nearby, helps him escape to safety.

Summary of the Fourth Observance

Cultivate an unshakable faith. Believe firmly in God, Gods, *guru* and your path to enlightenment. Trust in the words of the masters, the scriptures and traditions. Practice devotion and *sādhana* to inspire experiences that build advanced faith. Be loyal to your lineage, one with your *satguru.* Shun those who try to break your faith by argument and accusation. Avoid doubt and despair.

THE FOURTH OBSERVANCE

Faith

Āstikya आस्तिक्य

FAITH, *ĀSTIKYA,* IS THE FOURTH *NIYAMA.* FAITH IS A SUBSTANCE, A COLLECTION OF MOLECULES, MIND MOLECULES, EMOTION MOLECULES—AND SOME ARE EVEN PHYSIcal—collected together, charged with the energies of the Divine and the anxieties of the undivine, made into an astral form of shape, color and sound. Being a creation built up over time, faith can just as readily be destroyed, as the following phrases indicate: crisis of faith, loss of faith, dark night of the soul, and just plain confused disappointment leading to depression. Because of faith, groups of people are drawn together, cling together, remain together, intermarry and give birth, raising their children together in the substance of faith that their collective group is subconsciously committed to uphold.

Anyone can strengthen another's faith through encouragement, personal example, good natured humoring, praise, flattery, adulation, or take it away by the opposite methods. Many people with more faith than intellect are pawns in the hands of those who hold great faith, or of those who have little faith, or of those who have no faith at all. Therefore, we can see that a clear intellectual understanding of the philosophy is the bedrock to sustaining faith. Faith is on many levels and of many facets. We have faith in a person, a family, a system of government, science, astronomy, astrology. Faith in philosophy, religion, is the most tenuous and delicate kind and, we must say, the most rewarding of all faiths, because once it is sustained in unbroken continuity, the pure soul of the individual begins to shine forth.

Faith has eyes. It has three eyes. The seer who is looking at the world from the perspective of monistic Śaiva Siddhānta and sees clearly the final conclusions for all mankind has faith in his perception, because what he sees and has seen becomes stronger in his mind as the years go by. We have the faith of those who have two eyes upraised. They look at the seer as Dakshiṇāmūrti, God Himself, and gain strength from His every word. There is also the faith of those who have two eyes lowered. They are reading the scriptures, the teachings of all the seers, and building the aura of faith within their inner psyche. Then there are those who have faith with their eyes closed, blind faith. They know not, read not and are not thinking, but are entranced by the spiritual leader in whom they have faith as a personality. They are nodding their head up and down on his every word and when questioned are not able to adequately explain even one or two of his profound thoughts.

And then we have the others, who make up much of the world population today. They are also with eyes closed, but with heads down, shaking left and right, left and right. They see mostly the darker side of life. They are those who have no faith at all or suffer a semi-permanent loss of faith, who are disappointed in people, governments, systems, philosophies, religions. Their leaders they condemn. This is a sorry lot. Their home is the halls of depression, discouragement and confusion. Their upliftment is jealousy and anger.

Faith Is on Many Levels

Faith extends to another level, too, of pleasure for the sake of pleasure. Here we have the jet-set, the hedonists, the sensualists, the pornographers and their customers. All these groups have developed their own individual mindset and mix and interrelate among themselves, as the astral molecules of this amorphous substance of thought, emotion and belief that we call faith creates their attitudes toward the world, other people and their possessions.

The Hindu, therefore, is admonished by the *sapta ṛishis* themselves to believe firmly in God, Gods, *guru* and the path to enlightenment, lest he stray from the path of *dharma*—for faith is a powerful force. It can be given; it can be taken away. It is a national force, a community force, a group force, a family force. And it is more than that, as far as the Sanātana Dharma is concerned, which can be translated as the "eternal faith," the most strengthening and illuminating of all, for it gives courage to all to apply these twenty *yamas* and *niyamas*, which represent the final conclusions of the deepest deliverers of eternal wisdom who ever resided on this planet.

Some people have faith only when things are going right and lose faith when things go wrong. These are the ones who are looking up at their leaders, whom they really do not know, who are looking up at the scriptures, which they really do not understand. Because their eyes are closed, they are seeking to be sustained and constantly uplifted by others. "Do my *sādhana* for me" is their plea. And when some inconsistency arises or some expectation, unbeknownst to their leader and maybe never even recorded in the scriptures, does not manifest, a crisis of faith occurs. Then, more than often, they are off to another leader, another philosophy, to inevitably repeat the same experience. Devotees of this kind, who are called "groupies" in rock and roll, go from group to group, teacher to teacher, philosophy to philosophy. Fortunately for them, the rent is not expensive, the *bhajanas* are long and the food is good. The only embarrassing situation, which has to be manipulated, is the tactic of leaving one group without totally closing the door, and manipulatively opening the door of another group.

When that uplifted face with eyes closed has the spiritual experience of the eyes opening, the third eye flashing, he or she would have then found at last his or her *sampradāya*, traditional lineage of verbal teaching, and now be on the unshakable path. The molecules of faith have been converted and secured. They shall never turn back, because they have seen through the third eye the beginning and ending of the path, the traditional lineage ordained to carry them forth generation after generation. These souls become the articulate ones, masters of the philosophy. Their faith is so strong, they can share their molecules with others and mold others' faith molecules into traditional standards of the whys and wherefores that we all need on this planet, of how we should believe and think, where we go when we die, and all the eternal truths of the ultimate attainments of mankind.

Stages of Evolution

Faith is the intellect of the soul at its various stages of unfoldment. The soul comes forth from Lord Śiva as an embryo and progresses through three stages *(avasthā)* of existence: *kevala avasthā, sakala avasthā* and *śuddha avasthā.* During *kevala avasthā,* the soul is likened to a seed hidden in the ground or a spark of the Divine hidden in a cloud of unknowing called *āṇava,* the primal fetter of individuality, the first aspect of Lord Śiva's concealing grace, *tirodhāna śakti. Sakala avasthā,* the next stage in the soul's journey, is the period of bodily existence, the cyclic evolution through transmigration from body to body, under the additional powers of *māyā* and *karma,* the second and third aspects of the Lord's concealing grace.

The journey through *sakala avasthā* is also in three stages. The first is called *irul pāda,* "stage of darkness," where the soul's impetus is toward *pāśa-jñānam,* knowledge and experience of the world. The next period is *marul pāda,* "stage of confusion," where the soul begins to take account of its situation and finds itself caught between the world and God, not knowing which way to turn. This is called *paśu-jñānam,* the soul seeking to know its true nature. The last period is *arul pāda,* "stage of grace," when the soul yearns for the grace of

God. Now it has begun its true religious evolution with the constant aid of the Lord.

For the soul in darkness, *irul*, faith is primitive, illogical. In its childlike endeavors it clings to this faith. There is no intellect present in this young soul, only primitive faith and instinctive mind and body. But it is this faith in the unseen, the unknown, the words of the elders and its ability to adjust to community without ruffling everyone's feathers that matures the soul to the next *pāda—marul*, wherein faith becomes faith in oneself, close friends and associates, faith in one's intellectual remembrance of the opinions of others, even if they are wrong.

It is not very quickly that the soul gets out of this syndrome, because it is here that the *karmas* are made that bind the soul, surround the soul, the *karmas* of ignorance which must be gone through for the wisdom to emerge. Someone who is wise got that way by facing up to all the increments of ignorance. The *marul pāda* is very binding and tenacious, tenaciously binding. But as the external shell of *āṇava* is being built, the soul exercises itself in its own endeavor to break through. Its "still small voice" falls on deaf ears.

Yoga brings the soul into its next experiential pattern. The soul comes to find that if he performs good and virtuous deeds, life always seems to take a positive turn. Whereas in negative, unvirtuous acts he slowly becomes lost in a foreboding abyss of confusion. Thus, in faith, he turns toward the good and holy. A balance emerges in his life, called *iruvinaioppu.*

Whether he is conscious of it or not, he is bringing the three *malas—āṇava, karma* and *māyā*—under control. *Māyā* is less and less an enchanting temptress. *Karma* no longer controls his state of mind, tormenting him through battering experiences. And *āṇava*, his self-centered nature, is easing its hold, allowing him to feel a more universal compassion in life. This grows into a state called *malaparipakam*, the ripening of the *malas.*

This will allow, at the right moment in his life, *arul* to set in. This is known as the descent of grace, *śaktinipāta.* The internal descent is recognized as a tremendous yearning for Śiva. More and more, he wants to devote himself to all that is spiritual and holy. The outer descent of grace is the appearance of a *satguru.* There is no question as to who he is, for he sheds the same clear, spiritual vibration as that unknown something the soul feels emanating from his deepest self. It is when the soul has reached *malaparipakam* that the Lord's *tirodhāna* function, His concealing grace, has accomplished its work and gives way to *anugraha,* revealing grace, and the descent of grace, *śaktinipāta,* occurs.

At this stage, knowledge comes unbidden. Insights into human affairs are mere readings of past experiences, for those experiences that are being explained to others were actually lived through by the person himself. This is no mystery. It is the threshold of *śuddha avasthā.* Lord Śiva is at the top, Lord Gaṇeśa is at the bottom, and Lord Murugan is in the heart of it, in the center.

Faith in Tradition

The intellect in its capacity to contain truth is a very limited tool, while faith is a very broad, accommodating and embracing faculty. The mystery of life and beyond life, of Śiva, is really better understood through faith than through intellectual reasoning. The intellect is a memory/reason conglomerate from the lower *nāḍī/chakra* complex. Its refined ability to juggle information around is uncanny in some instances. Nevertheless, the intellect is built upon what we hear and remember, what we experience and remember, what we explain to others who are refined or gross in reasoning faculties. What we remember of it all and the portions that have been forgotten may be greatly beneficial to those listening, or it may be confusing, but it is certainly not Truth with a capital "T."

There are two kinds of faith. The first kind is faith in those masters, adepts, *yogīs* and *ṛishis* who have had similar experiences and have spoken about them in similar ways, unedited by the ignorant. We, therefore, can have faith that some Truth was revealed from within themselves, from some deep, inner or higher source. The second aspect of faith is in one's own spiritual, unsought-for, unbidden flashes of intuition, revelations or visions, which one remembers even stronger as the months go by, more vividly than something read from a book, seen on television or heard from a friend or a philosopher. These personal revelations create a new, superconscious intellect when verified by what *yogīs* and *ṛishis* and the *sādhus* have seen and heard and whose explanations centuries have preserved. These are the old souls of the *śuddha avasthā,* being educated from within out, building a new intellect from superconscious insights. Their faith is unshakable, undaunted, for it is themself. It is just who they are at this stage of the evolution, the maturation, of their soul in the *śuddha avasthā.*

One of the aspects of faith is the acceptance of tradition rather than the questioning or doubting of traditions. Another is trust in the process of spiritual unfoldment, so that when one is going through an experience, one always believes that the process is happening, instead of thinking that today's negative experience is outside the process. However, it is not possible for souls in the *irul pāda,* stage of darkness, to trust in the process of anything except their need for food, a few bodily comforts and their gaining the abilities to adjust transparently into a community without committing too many crimes for which they would be severely punished. They gain their lessons through the action-and-painful-reaction ways.

It is difficult and nearly impossible for those in the *marul pāda,* stage of confusion, to have faith in the process of spiritual unfoldment and trust in tradition, because they are developing their personal ego, manufacturing *karmas,* good, bad and mixed, to sustain their physical existence for hundreds of lives. They will listen to sermons with a deaf ear and, after they are over, enjoy the food and the idle chatter the most. They will read books on philosophy and rationalize their teachings as relevant only to the past. The great knowledge of the past tradition, even the wisdom their grandparents might hold, is an encroachment on their proud sovereignty.

It is only when the soul reaches the maturity to enter the *arul pāda,* the stage of grace, that the ability will come from within to lean on the past and on tradition, perform the present *sādhanas,* live within *dharma* and carve a future for themselves and others by bringing the best of the past, which is tradition, forward into the future. This transition is a happy one. Truth now has a capital "T" and is always told. The restraints, the *yamas,* truly have been perfected and are a vital part of the DNA system of individual living beings. Now, as he enters the *arul pāda,* the *niyamas,* spiritual practices, stand out strongly in his mind.

The Sanskrit word *āstikya* means "that which is," or "that which exists." Thus, for Hindus *faith* means believing in what is. *Āstikya* refers to one who believes in what is, one who is pious and faithful. We can see that these two words, *faith* and *āstikya,* are similar in nature. Faith is the spiritual-intellectual mind, developed through many superconscious insights blended together through cognition, not through reason. The insights do not have to be remembered, because they are firmly impressed as *saṁskāras* within the inner mind.

There is an old saying favored by practical, experiential intellectuals, "Seeing is believing." A more profound adage is "Believing is seeing." The scientists and the educators of today live in the *marul pāda.* They see with their two eyes and pass judgments based on what they currently believe.

The *ṛishis* of the past and the *ṛishis* of the now and those yet to come in the future also are seers. There is a thin thread through the history of China, Japan, India, England and all of Europe, Africa, the Americas, Polynesia and all the countries of the world connecting seers and what they have seen. This seeing is not with the two eyes. It is with the third eye, the eye of the soul. One cannot erase through argument or coercion that which has been seen. The seer relates his seeing to the soul of the one who hears. This is *sampradāya.* This is *guru-śishya* transference. This is Truth. This is *śuddha.* This is the end of this *upadeśa.*

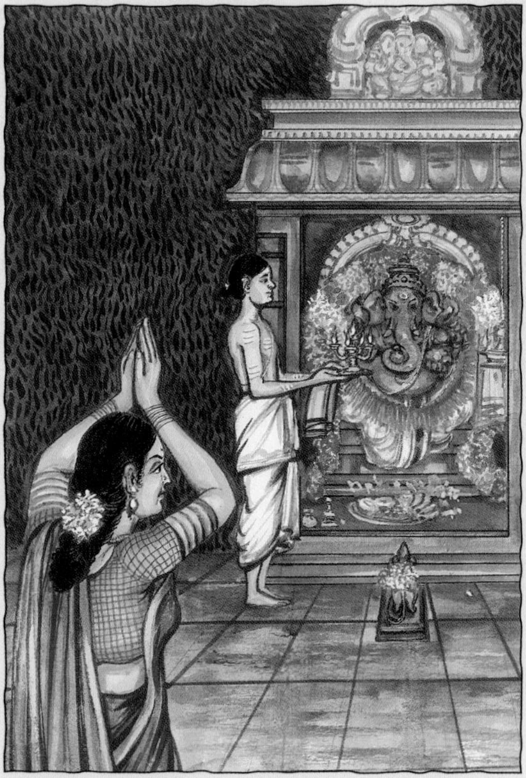

Hands raised in adoration during a pūjā, *a devotee venerates Gaṇeśa in an act of* Īśvarapūjana, *worship.*

Summary of the Fifth Observance

Cultivate devotion through daily worship and meditation. Set aside one room of your home as God's shrine. Offer fruit, flowers or food daily. Learn a simple *pūjā* and the chants. Meditate after each *pūjā.* Visit your shrine before and after leaving the house. Worship in heartfelt devotion, clearing the inner channels to God, Gods and *guru* so their grace flows toward you and loved ones.

THE FIFTH OBSERVANCE

Worship

Īśvarapūjana ईश्वरपूजन

WORSHIP, ĪŚVARAPŪJANA, IS THE FIFTH *NIYAMA*. LET US DECLARE, IN THE LAST ANALYSIS, THAT HUMAN LIFE IS EITHER WORSHIP OR WARSHIP, HIGHER NATURE OR LOWER NATURE. We need say no more. But we will. The brief explanation for Īśvarapūjana is to cultivate devotion through daily worship and meditation. The soul's evolution from its conception is based solely on Īśvarapūjana, the return to the source. In the *irul pāda,* the stage of darkness, its return to the source is more imminent than actual. The burning desire is there, driven by the instinctive feelings and emotions of living within the seven *chakras* below the *mūlādhāra.* There is a natural seeking on the way up. People here will worship almost anything to get out of this predicament. Bound in blind faith, with the absence of a coherent intellect guided by reason, and the absence of a matured intellect developed by superconscious experience, they struggle out of their shell of ignorance, through worship, to a better life. The small thread of intuition keeps assuring them it is there, within their reach if they but strive. They call God, they fear God, seek to be close to Him and see Him as oh-so-far away.

When they are matured and stepping into adolescence in the *marul pāda*, where confusion prevails, worship and the trappings and traditions that go with it seem to be primitive, unreasonable and can all well be dispensed with. It is here that a young lady looks into the mirror and says, "What a fine person! I am more beautiful than all the other girls I know." A young man may likewise be conceited about his looks or physique. Worship still exists, but is tied closely to narcissism. It is only in the stage of grace, *arul,* and on its doorstep that true worship arises, which is invoking and opening up to the great beings, God, Gods and *devas,* in order to commune with them.

Faith, *āstikya,* creates the attitudes for the action of worship. We can see that from the soul's conception to its fullness of maturity into the final merger with God Śiva Himself, worship, communication, looking up, blending with, is truly monistic Śaiva Siddhānta, the final conclusions for all mankind. We can conclude that in Sanātana Dharma faith is in What Is, and in the Abrahamic religions faith is in What Is Yet to Be.

Worship could be defined as communication on a very high level: a truly sophisticated form of "channeling," as New-Age people might say; clairvoyant or clairaudient experience, as mystics would describe it; or heart-felt love interchanged between Deity and devotee, as the ordinary person would describe it. Worship for the Hindu is on many levels and of many kinds. In the home, children worship their father and mother as God and Goddess because they love them. The husband worships his wife as a Goddess. The wife worships her husband as a God. In the shrine room, the entire family together worships images of Gods, Goddesses and saints, beseeching them as their dear friends. The family goes to the temple daily, or at least once a week, attends seasonal festivals and takes a far-off pilgrimage once a year. Worship is the binding force that keeps the Hindu family together. On a deeper level, external worship is internalized, worshiping God within through meditation and contemplation. This form of worship leads into *yoga* and profound mystical experiences.

Rites of Worship

Many people are afraid to do *pūjā,* specific, traditional rites of worship, because they feel they don't have enough training or don't understand the mystical principles behind it well enough. To this concern I would say that the priesthood in Hinduism is sincere, devout and dedicated. Most Hindus depend on the priests to perform the *pūjās* and sacraments for them, or to train them to perform home *pūjā* and give them permission to do so through initiation, called *dīkshā*. However, simple *pūjās* may be performed by anyone wishing to invoke grace from God, Mahādevas and *devas*.

Love and dedication and the outpouring from the highest *chakras* of spiritual energies of the lay devotee are often greater than any professional priest could summon within himself. Devotees of this caliber have come up in Hindu society throughout the ages with natural powers to invoke the Gods and manifest in the lives of temple devotees many wondrous miracles.

There is also an informal order of priests called *paṇḍara*, which is essentially the self-appointed priest who is accepted by the community to perform *pūjās* at a sacred tree, a simple shrine or an abandoned temple. He may start with the *mantra Aum* and learn a few more *mantras* as he goes along. His efficaciousness can equal that of the most advanced Sanskrit *śāstrī*, performing in the grandest temple. Mothers, daughters, aunts, fathers, sons, uncles, all may perform *pūjā* within their own home, and do, as the Hindu home is considered to be nothing less than an extension of the nearby temple. In the Hindu religion, unlike the Western religions, there is no one who stands between man and God.

Years ago, in the late 1950s, I taught beginning seekers how to offer the minimal, simplest form of *pūjā* at a simple altar with fresh water, flowers, a small candle, incense, a bell and a stone. This brings together the four elements, earth, air, fire and water—and your own mind is *ākāśa*, the fifth element. The liturgy is simply chanting "Aum." This is the generic *pūjā* which anyone can do before proper initiation comes from the right sources. People of any religion can perform Hindu *pūjā* in this way.

All Hindus have guardian *devas* who live on the astral plane and guide, guard and protect their lives. The great Mahādevas in the temple that the devotees frequent send their *deva* ambassadors into the homes to live with the devotees. A room is set aside for these permanent unseen guests, a room that the whole family can enter and sit in and commune inwardly with these refined beings who are dedicated to protecting the family generation after generation. Some of them are their own ancestors. A token shrine in a bedroom or a closet or a niche in a kitchen is not enough to attract these Divinities. One would not host an honored guest in one's closet or have him or her sleep in the kitchen and expect the guest to feel welcome, appreciated, loved. All Hindus are taught from childhood that the guest is God, and they treat any guest royally who comes to visit. Hindus also treat God as God and *devas* as Gods when they come to live permanently in the home.

But liberal sects of Hinduism teach that God and *devas* are only figments of one's imagination. These sects are responsible for producing a more materialistic and superficial group of followers. Not so the deep, mystical Hindu, who dedicates his home to God and sets a room aside for God. To him and the family, they are moving into God's house and living with God. Materialistic, superficial Hindus feel that God *might* be living, sometimes, maybe, in their house. Their homes are fraught with confusion, deceptive dealings, back-biting, anger, even rage, and their marriages nowadays often end in divorce.

They and all those who live in the lower nature are restricted from performing *pūjā,* because when and if they do *pūjā,* the invocation calls up the demons rather than calling down the *devas.* The *asuric* beings invoked into the home by angry people, and into the temple by angry priests, or by contentious, argumentative, sometimes rageful boards of directors, take great satisfaction in creating more confusion and escalating simple misunderstandings into arguments leading to angry words, hurt feelings and more. With this in mind, once anger is experienced, thirty-one days should pass to close the door on the *chakras* below the *mūlādhāra* before *pūjā* may again be performed by that individual. Simple waving of incense before the icons is permissible, but not the passing of flames, ringing of bells or the chanting of any *mantra,* other than the simple recitation of *Aum.*

Living in God's Home

The ideal of Īśvarapūjana, worship, is to always be living with God, living with Śiva, in God's house, which is also your house, and regularly going to God's temple. This lays the foundation for finding God within. How can someone find God within if he doesn't live in God's house as a companion to God in his daily life? The answer is obvious. It would only be a theoretical pretense, based mainly on egoism. If one really believes that God is in his house, what kinds of attitudes does this create? First of all, since family life is based around food, the family would feed God in His own room at least three times a day, place the food lovingly before His picture, leave, close the door and let God and His *devas* eat in peace. God and the *devas* do enjoy the food, but they do so by absorbing the *prāṇas,* the energies, of the food. When the meal is over, and after the family has eaten, God's plates are picked up, too. What is left on God's plate is eaten as *prasāda,* as a blessing. God should be served as much as the hungriest member of the family, not just a token amount. Of course, God, Gods and the *devas* do not always remain in the shrine room. They wander freely throughout the house, listening to and observing the entire family, guests and friends. Since the family is living in God's house, and God is not living in *their* house, the voice of God is easily heard as their conscience.

When we are living in God's house, it is easy to see God as pure energy and life within every living form, the trees, the flowers, the plants, the fire, the Earth, humans, animals and all creatures. When we see this life, which is manifest most in living beings, we are seeing God Śiva. Many families are too selfish to set aside a room for God. Though they have their personal libraries, rumpus rooms, two living rooms, multiple bedrooms, their superficial religion borders on a new Indian religion. Their shrine is a closet, or pictures of God and Goddesses on the vanity mirror of their dressing table. The results of such worship are nil, and their life reflects the chaos that we see in the world today.

The psychology and the decision and the religion is, "Do we live with God, or does God occasionally visit us?" Who is the authority in the home, an unreligious, ignorant, domineering elder? Or is it God Śiva Himself, or Lord Murugan or Lord Gaṇeśa, whom the entire family, including elders, bow down to because they have resigned themselves to the fact that they are living in the *āśrama* of Mahādevas? This is religion. This is Īśvarapūjana.

It is often said that worship is not only a performance at a certain time of day in a certain place, but a state of being in which every act, morning to night, is done in Śiva consciousness, in which life becomes an offering to God. Then we can begin to see Śiva in everyone we meet. When we try, just try—and we don't have to be successful all the time—to separate the life of the individual from his personality, immediately we are in higher consciousness and can reflect contentment and faith, compassion, steadfastness and all the higher qualities, which is sometimes not possible to do if we are only looking at the external person. This practice, of Īśvarapūjana *sādhana,* can be performed all through the day and even in one's dreams at night.

Meditation, too, in the Hindu way is based on worship. It is true that Hindus do teach meditation techniques to those who have Western backgrounds as a mind-manipulative experience. However, a Hindu adept, *ṛishi* or *jñānī*, even an experienced elder, knows that meditation is a natural outgrowth of the *charyā, kriyā* and *yoga* paths. It is based on a religious foundation, as trigonometry is based on geometry, algebra and arithmetic.

If you are worshiping properly, if you take worship to its pinnacle, you are in perfect meditation. We have seen many devotees going through the form of worship with no communication with the God they are worshiping or even the stone that the God uses as a temporary body. They don't even have a smile on their face. They are going through the motions because they have been taught that meditation is the ultimate, and worship can be dispensed with after a certain time. Small wonder that when they are in meditation, their minds are confused and subconscious overloads harass them. Breathing is irregular, and if made regular has to be forced. Their materialistic outlook on life—of seeing God everywhere, yet not in those places they rationalize God can never possibly be—contradicts their professed dedication to the Hindu way of life.

Yes, truly, worship unreservedly. Perfect this. Then, after initiation, internalize that worship through *yoga* practices given by a *satguru.* Through that same internal worship, unreservedly, you will eventually attain the highest goal. These are the Śaiva Siddhānta conclusions of the seven *ṛishis* who live within the *sahasrāra chakra* of all souls.

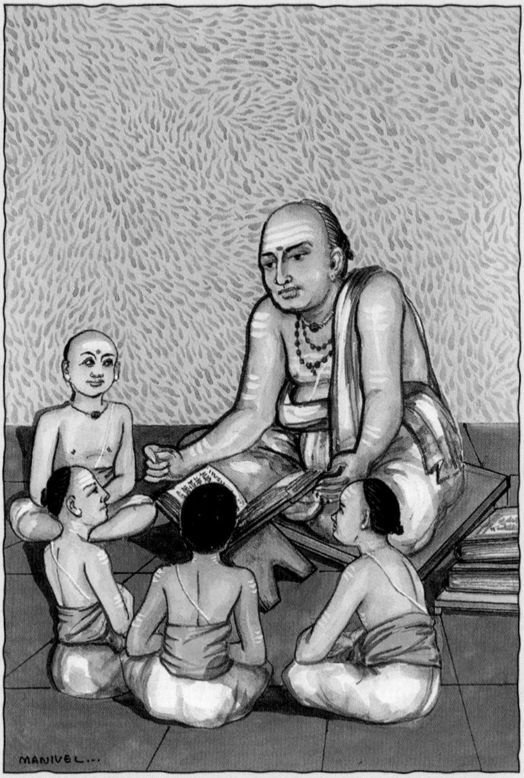

A teacher passes along the gift of scriptural learning to four boys through recitation of holy scriptural texts.

Summary of the Sixth Observance

Eagerly hear the scriptures, study the teachings and listen to the wise of your lineage. Choose a *guru,* follow his path and don't waste time exploring other ways. Read, study and, above all, listen to readings and dissertations by which wisdom flows from knower to seeker. Avoid secondary texts that preach violence. Revere and study the revealed scriptures, the *Vedas* and *Āgamas.*

THE SIXTH OBSERVANCE

Scriptural Study

Siddhānta Śravaṇa सिद्धान्तश्रवण

S*IDDHĀNTA ŚRAVAṆA*, SCRIPTURAL STUDY, THE SIXTH *NIYAMA*, IS THE END OF THE SEARCH. PRIOR TO THIS END, PRIOR TO FINDING THE *SATGURU*, WE ARE FREE TO STUDY ALL THE scriptures of the world, of all religions, relate and interrelate them in our mind, manipulate their meanings and justify their final conclusions. We are free to study all of the sects and *sampradāyas*, all denominations, lineages and teachings, everything under the banner of Hinduism—the Śaivites, the Vaishṇavites, the Smārtas, Gaṇapatis, Ayyappans, Śāktas and Murugans and their branches.

Scriptures within Hinduism are voluminous. The methods of teaching are awesome in their multiplicity. As for teachers, there is one on every corner in India. Ask a simple question of an elder, and he is duty-bound to give a lengthy response from the window he is looking out of, opened by the *sampradāya* he or his family has subscribed to, maybe centuries ago, of one or another sect within this great pantheon we call Hinduism.

Before we come to the fullness of *siddhānta śravaṇa*, we are also free to investigate psychologies, psychiatries, pseudo-sciences, ways of behavior of the human species, existentialism, humanism, secular humanism, materialism and the many other modern "-isms," which are so multitudinous and still multiplying. Their spokesmen are many. Libraries are full of them. All the "-isms" and "-ologies" are there, and they beckon, hands outstretched to receive, to seduce, sometimes even seize, the seeker. The seeker on the path of *siddhānta śravaṇa* who is at least relatively successful at the ten restraints must make a choice. He knows he has to. He knows he must. He has just entered the consciousness of the *mūlādhāra chakra* and is becoming steadfast on the upward climb.

Have full faith that when your *guru* does appear, after you have made yourself ready through the ten restraints and the first five practices, you will know in every nerve current of your being that this is your guide on the path through the next five practices: 1) *siddhānta śravaṇa,* scriptural study—following one verbal lineage and not pursuing any others; 2) *mati,* cognition—developing a spiritual will and intellect with a *guru's* guidance; 3) *vrata,* sacred vows—fulfilling religious vows, rules, and observances faithfully; 4) *japa,* recitation of holy *mantras*—here we seek initiation from the *guru* to perform this practice; and 5) *tapas,* performing austerity, *sādhana,* penance and sacrifice, also under the *guru's* guidance.

Siddhānta śravaṇa is a discipline, an ancient traditional practice in *satguru* lineages, to carry the devotee from one *chakra* in consciousness to another. Each *sampradāya* defends its own teachings and principles against other *sampradāyas* to maintain its pristine purity and admonishes followers from investigating any of them. Such exploration of other texts should all be done before seeking to fulfill *siddhānta śravaṇa.* Once under the direction of and having been accepted by a *guru,* any further delving into extraneous doctrines would be disapproved and disallowed.

Siddhānta śravaṇa is more than just focusing on a single doctrine. It is developing through scriptural study an entirely new mind fabric, subconsciously and consciously, which will entertain an explanation for all future *prārabdha karmas* and *karmas* created in this life to be experienced for the duration of the physical life of the disciple. *Siddhānta śravaṇa* is even more. It lays the foundation for initiation within the fabric of the nerve system of the disciple. Even more, it portrays any differences in his thinking, the *guru's* thought, the *sampradāya's* principles, philosophy and underlying practices.

Transmitting Tradition

Siddhānta śravaṇa literally means "scriptural listening." It is one thing to read the *Vedas, Upanishads* and *Yoga Sūtras,* but it is quite another to hear their teachings from one who knows, because it is through hearing that the transmission of subtle knowledge occurs, from knower to seeker. And that is why listening is preferred over intellectual study.

Because sound is the first creation, knowledge is transferred through sound of all kinds. It is important that one listen to the highest truths of a *sampradāya* from one who has realized them. The words, of course, will be familiar. They have been read by the devotee literally hundreds of times, but to hear them from the mouth of the enlightened *ṛishi* is to absorb his unspoken realization, as he re-realizes his realization while he reads them and speaks them out. This is Śaiva Siddhānta. This is true *sampradāya*—thought, meaning and knowledge conveyed through words spoken by one who has realized the Ultimate. The words will be heard, the meaning the *satguru* understands as meaning will be absorbed by the subconscious mind of the devotee, and the superconscious, intuitive knowledge will impress the subsuperconscious mind of the devotees who absorb it, who milk it out of the *satguru* himself. This and only this changes the life pattern of the devotee. There is no other way. This is why one must come to the *guru* open, like a child, ready and willing to absorb, and to go through many tests. And this is why one must choose one's *guru* wisely and be ready for such an event in one's life.

Sampradāya actually means an orally transmitted tradition, unwritten and unrecorded in any other way. True, *satgurus* of *sampradāyas* do write books nowadays, make tape recordings, videos and correspond. This is mini-*sampradāya,* the bud of a flower before opening, the shell of an egg before the bird hatches and flies off, the cocoon before the butterfly emerges. This is mini-*sampradāya*—just a taste, but it does lay a foundation within the *śishya's* mind of who the *guru* is, what he thinks, what he represents, the beginning and ending of his path, the *sampradāya* he represents, carries forth and is bound to carry forth to the next generation, the next and the next. But really potent *sampradāya* is listening, actually listening to the *guru's* words, his explanations. It stimulates thought. Once-remembered words take on new meanings. Old knowledge is burnt out and replaced with new. This is *sampradāya.*

Are you ready for a *satguru?* Perhaps not. When you are ready, and he comes into your life through a dream, a vision or a personal meeting, the process begins. The devotee takes one step toward the *guru*—a simple meeting, a simple dream. The *guru* is bound to take nine steps toward the devotee, not ten, not eleven or twelve, only nine, and then wait for the devotee to take one more step. Then another nine ensue. This is the dance. This is *sampradāya.*

When a spiritual experience comes, a real awakening of light, a flash of realization, a knowing that has never been seen in print, or if it had been is long-since forgotten, it gives great courage to the devotee to find that it had already been experienced and written about by others within his chosen *sampradāya.*

If all the temples were destroyed, the *gurus* would come forth and rebuild them. If all the scriptures were destroyed, the *ṛishis* would reincarnate and rewrite them. If all the *gurus, swāmīs, ṛishis, sādhus,* saints and sages were systematically destroyed, they would take births here and there around the globe and continue as if nothing had ever happened. So secure is the Eternal Truth on the planet, so unshakable, that it forges ahead undaunted through the mouths of many. It forges ahead undaunted through the temples' open doors. It forges ahead undaunted in scriptures now lodged in nearly every library in the world. It forges ahead undaunted, mystically hidden from the unworthy, revealed only to the worthy, who restrain themselves by observing some or all of the *yamas* and who practice a few *niyamas.*

Coming under a *satguru* of one lineage, all scripture, temple and home tradition may be taken away from the eyes of the experience of the newly accepted devotee. In another tradition, scripture may be taken away and temple worship allowed to remain, so that only the words of the *guru* are heard. In still another tradition, the temple, the scripture and the voice of the *guru* are always there—but traditionally only the scripture which has the approval of the *satguru* and is totally in accord with his principles, practices and the underlying philosophy of the *sampradāya.*

Living One Path Perfectly

Life is long; there are apparently many years ahead. But time is short. One never knows when he is going to die. The purpose of *sampradāya* is to restrict and narrow down, to reach out to an attainable goal. We must not consider our life and expected longevity as giving us the time and permission to do investigative comparisons of one *sampradāya* to another. This may be done before making up one's mind to follow a traditional verbal lineage. After that, pursuing other paths, even in passing, would be totally unacceptable.

But it is also totally unacceptable to assume the attitude of denigration of other paths, or to assume the attitude that "our way is the only way." There are fourteen currents in the *sushumṇā.* Each one is a valid way to escalate consciousness into the *chakra* at the top of the skull and beyond. And at every point in time, there is a living *guru,* possessing a physical body, ordained to control one or more of these *nāḍīs,* currents, within the *sushumṇā.* All are valid paths. One should not present itself as superseding another. Let here be no mistake about this.

The *yamas* and *niyamas* are the core of Hindu disciplines and restraints for individuals, groups, communities and nations. In fact, they outline various stages of the path in the development of the soul, leading out of the *marul pāda* into the *arul pāda,* from confusion into grace, leading to the feet of the *satguru,* as the last five practices indicate—*siddhānta śravaṇa, mati, vrata, japa* and *tapas.*

Since the *sampradāyas* are all based on Hinduism, which is based on the *Vedas,* any teacher of Indian spirituality who rejects the *Vedas* is therefore not a Hindu and should not be considered as such. Anybody in his right mind will be able to accept the last section of the *Vedas,* the *Upanishads,* and see the truth therein. One at least has to accept that as the basis of *siddhānta śravaṇa.* If even that is rejected, we must consider the teacher a promulgator of a new Indian religion, neo-American religion, neo-European religion, neo-New-Age religion, nonreligion, neo-*sannyāsī* religion, or some other "neo-ism" or "neo-ology." This is not *sampradāya.* This is not *siddhānta śravaṇa.* This is what we speak against. These are not the eternal paths. Why? Because they have not been tried and tested. They are not based on traditional lineages; nor have they survived the ravages of time, changing societies, wars, famine and the infiltration of ignorance.

For *sādhakas, yogīs, swāmīs* and mendicants who have freed themselves from the world, permanently or for a period of time according to their vows, these *yamas* and *niyamas* are not only restraints and practices, but mandatory controls. They are not only practices, but obligatory disciplines, and once performed with this belief and attitude, they will surely lead the mendicant to his chosen goal, which can only be the height that his *prārabdha karmas* in this life permit, unless those *karmas* are burned out under extreme *tapas* under the guidance of a *satguru.*

Some might still wonder, why limit oneself to listening to scripture of one particular lineage, especially if it has been practically memorized? The answer is that what has been learned must be experienced personally, and experience comes in many depths. This is the purpose of disregarding or rejecting all other *sampradāyas,* -ism's, -ologies and sects, or denominations, and of limiting scriptural listening to just one *sampradāya,* so that each subtle increment of the divine truths amplified within it is realized through personal experience. This and only this—experience, realization, illumination—can be carried on to the next birth. What one has merely memorized is not transforming and is forgotten perhaps shortly after death. Let there be no mistake that *siddhānta śravaṇa,* scriptural listening, is the only way; and when the seeker is ready, the *guru* will appear and enter his life.

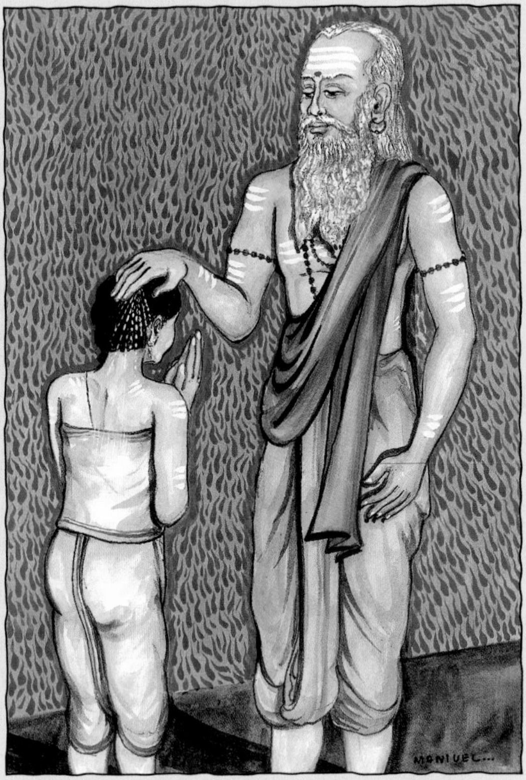

A sage blesses a young boy, bestowing upon him mati, *insightful cognition and spiritual understanding.*

Summary of the Seventh Observance

Develop a spiritual will and intellect with your *satguru's* guidance. Strive for knowledge of God, to awaken the light within. Discover the hidden lesson in each experience to develop a profound understanding of life and yourself. Through meditation, cultivate intuition by listening to the still, small voice within, by understanding the subtle sciences, inner worlds and mystical texts.

THE SEVENTH OBSERVANCE

Cognition

Mati मति

COGNITION, *MATI,* IS THE SEVENTH *NIYAMA.* COGNITION MEANS UNDERSTANDING; BUT DEEPER THAN UNDERSTANDING, IT IS SEEING THROUGH TO THE OTHER SIDE OF THE results that a thought, a word or an action would have in the future, before the thought, word or action has culminated. *Mati* is the development of a spiritual will and intellect through the grace of a *satguru,* an enlightened master. *Mati* can only come this way. It is a transference of divine energies from the *satguru* to the *śishya,* building a purified intellect honed down by the *guru* for the *śishya,* and a spiritual will developed by the *śishya* by following the religious *sādhanas* the *guru* has laid down until the desired results are attained to the *guru's* satisfaction. *Sādhana* is always done under a *guru's* direction. This is the worthy *sādhana* that bears fruit.

Mati, cognition, on a higher level is the awakening of the third eye, looking out through the heart *chakra,* seeing through the *māyā,* the interacting creation, preservation and dissolution of the molecules of matter. *Mati* is all this and more, for within each one who is guided by the *guru's* presence lies the ability to see not only with the two eyes but with all three simultaneously. The spiritual intellect described herein is none other than wisdom, or a "wise dome," if you will. Wisdom is the timely application of knowledge, not merely the opinions of others, but knowledge gained through deep observation.

The *guru's* guidance is supreme in the life of the dedicated devotee who is open for training. The verbal lineages of the many *sampradāyas* have withstood the tests of time, turmoil, decay and ravage of external hostility. The *sampradāyas* that have sustained man and lifted him above the substratum of ignorance are actually great nerve currents within the *sushumṇā* of the awakened *satguru* himself. To go further on the path of *yoga,* one will encounter within his own *sushumṇā* current—within one of the fourteen *nāḍīs* within it—a *satguru,* a *guru* who preaches Truth. He will meet this *guru* in a dream or in his physical body, and through the *guru's* grace and guidance will be allowed to continue the upward climb. These fourteen currents, at every point in time on the surface of the Earth, have a *satguru* attached to them, ready and waiting to open the portals of the beyond into the higher *chakras,* the throat, the third eye and the cranium.

To say, "I have awakened my throat *chakra,*" "I now live in my third eye" or "I am developing my *sahasrāra chakra,*" without being able to admit to being under a *guru,* a *satguru* who knows and is personally directing the devotee, is foolishness, a matter of imagination. It is in the heart *chakra,* the *chakra* of cognition, that seekers see through the veils of ignorance, illusion, *māyā's* interacting preservation, creation and destruction, and gain a unity with and love for the universe—all those within it, creatures, peoples and all the various forms—feeling themselves a part of it.

Here, on this threshold of the *anāhata chakra,* there are two choices. One is following the *sampradāya* of a *satguru* for the next upward climb into the *viśuddha, ājñā* and *sahasrāra.* The other is remaining *guru-less,* becoming one's own *guru,* and possibly delving into various forms of psychism, astrology, some forms of modern science, psychic crime-detection, tarot cards, pendulums, crystal gazing, psychic healing, past-life reading or fortunetelling. These psychic abilities, when developed, can be an impediment, a deterrent, a barrier, a Berlin Wall to future spiritual development. They develop the *āṇava,* the ego, and are the first renunciations the *satguru* would ask a devotee to make prior to being accepted.

Coming under a *satguru*, one performs according to the *guru's* direction with full faith and confidence. This is why scriptures say a *guru* must be carefully chosen, and when one is found, to follow him with all your heart, to obey and fulfill his every instruction better than he would have expected you to, and most importantly, even better than you would have expected of yourself.

Psychic abilities are not in themselves deterrents on the path. They are permitted to develop later, after Paraśiva, *nirvikalpa samādhi*, has been attained and fully established within the individual. But this, too, would be under the *guru's* grace and guidance, for these abilities are looked at as tools to fulfill certain works assigned by the *guru* to the devotee to fulfill until the end of the life of the physical body.

It is the personal ego, the *āṇava*, that is developed through the practice of palmistry, astrology, tarot cards, fortunetelling, past-life reading, crystal gazing, crystal healing, *prāṇa* transference, etc., etc., etc. This personal ego enhancement is a gift from those who are healed, who are helped, who are encouraged and who are in awe of the psychic power awakened in the heart *chakra* of this most perfect person of the higher consciousness who doesn't anger, display fear or exhibit any lower qualities.

Untying the Bonds

The three *malas* that bind us are: *māyā*, the ever-perpetuating dance of creation, preservation and dissolution; *karma* (our *prārabdha karma*, brought with us to face in this life, along with the *karma* we are creating now and will create in the future); and *āṇava*, the ego, ignorance or sense of separateness. *Māyā* can be understood, seen through and adjusted to through the heart-*chakra* powers of cognition, contentment and compassion. *Karmas* can be harnessed through regular forms of disciplinary practices of body, mind and emotions, and the understanding of the law of *karma* itself as a force that is sent out through thought, feeling and action and most often returns to us through other peoples' thought, feeling and action. But it is the *āṇava mala,* the *mala* of personal ego, that is the binding chain which cannot be so easily dealt with. It is the last to go. It is only at the point of death, before the greatest *mahāsamādhi* of the greatest *ṛishi,* that the *āṇava mala* chain is finally broken.

If we compare this *āṇava mala,* personal ego, to an actual *mālā,* a string of *rudrāksha* beads, the purpose on the path at this stage, of *mati,* is to begin eliminating the beads, making the chain shorter and shorter. The *mālā* should be getting shorter and shorter rather than our adding beads to it so that it gets longer and longer. A warning: if the *āṇava mala*—symbolically a garland of *rudrāksha* beads—has thirty-six beads and it steadily grows to 1,008 because of practices and the adulation connected with them within the psychic realms of the pseudoscience of parapsychology—such as bending spoons, telepathy, channeling and ectoplasmic manifestations—this 1,008 strand of *rudrāksha* beads could become so heavy, so dangerous to the wearer, that eventually he would trip and fall on his nose. The wise say, "Pride goes before a fall." And the still wiser know that "spiritual pride is the most difficult pride to deal with, to eliminate, to rise above in a lifetime." The spiritually proud never open themselves to a *satguru.* The mystically humble do.

Mati has also been interpreted as "good intellect, acute intelligence, a mind directed toward right knowledge, or Vedic knowledge." Good intellect, in the context of a Hindu seer, would be right knowledge based on *siddhānta śravaṇa,* scriptural study. Acute intelligence, of course, means "see-through" or panoramic intelligence which cognizes the entire picture rather than only being aware of one of its parts. "A mind directed toward right knowledge or Vedic knowledge" refers to the intellect developed through *siddhānta śravaṇa.* The study of the *Vedas* and other scriptures purifies the intellect, as belief creates attitude, and attitude creates action. An intellect based on truths of the Sanātana Dharma is intelligent to the divine laws of the universe and harnessed into fulfilling them as a part of it. To this end, all the *prārabdha karmas* of this life and the action-reaction conglomerates formed in this life are directed. The intellect, like the emotions, is a force, disciplined or undisciplined, propelled by right knowledge or wrong knowledge. It, of itself, processes, logically or illogically, both kinds of knowledge or their mix. What harnesses the intellect is *siddhānta śravaṇa,* study of the teachings and listening to the wise of an established, traditional lineage that has stood the test of time, ravage and all attempts at conversion.

The intellect is a neutral tool which can be used for bad or for good purposes. But unlike the emotions, which are warm, and also neutral, the intellect is cold. It is the fire of the *kuṇḍalinī* force—impregnating the intellect, purifying it, burning out the ignorance of wrong concepts, thought forms, beliefs, connected attitudes, causing an aversion to certain actions—that forges the purified intellect and spiritual will of cognition, known as *mati. Mati,* in summary, is the harnessing of the intellect by the soul to live a spiritual life.

Purifying the Intellect

There are many things which have their claim on people's minds. For many it is the physical body. The hypochondriac thinks about it all the time. Then there is the employer who has bought the intellect of the employee. The emotions consume the intellect with hurt feelings and the rhetorical questions that ensue, elated feelings and the continued praise that is expected. And then there is television, the modern *viśvaguru* that guides the intellect into confusion. As a dream leads only to waking up, television leads only to turning it off. Yes, there are many things that claim the intellect, many more than we have spoken about already.

The intellect is guided by the physical; the intellect is guided by the emotions, by other people, and by mechanical devices. And the intellect is guided by the intellect itself, like a computer processing and reprocessing knowledge without really understanding any of it. It is at the stage when anger has subsided, jealousy is unacceptable behavior and fear is a distant feeling, when memory is intact, the processes of reason are working well, the willpower is strong and the integrity is stable, when one is looking out from the *anāhata chakra* window of consciousness, when instinctive-intellectual thought meets the superconscious of the *purusha,* the soul, that the inner person lays claim on the outer person.

There is a struggle, to be sure, as the "I Am" struggles to take over the "was then." It's simple. The last *mala,* the *āṇava "mālā,"* has to start losing its beads. The personal ego must go for universal cosmic identity, Satchidānanda, to be maintained. This, then, is the platform of the throat *chakra,* the *viśuddha chakra,* of a true, all-pervasive, never-relenting spiritual identity. Here *guru* and *śishya* live in oneness in divine communication. Even if never a word is spoken, the understanding in the devotee begins to grow and grow and grow.

Some people think of the intellect as informing the superconscious or soul nature, instructing or educating it. Some people even think that they can command the Gods to do their bidding. These are the people that also think that their wife is a slave, that children are their servants, and who cleverly deceive their employers and governments through learned arts of deception.

These are the prototypes of the well-developed ignorant person, even though he might feign humility and proclaim religiousness. It is the religion that he professes, if he keeps doing so, that will pull him out of this darkness. When the first beam of light comes through the *mūlādhāra chakra,* he will start instructing his own soul as to what it should do for him, yet he still habitually dominates his wife, inhibiting her own feelings as a woman, and his children, inhibiting their feelings in experiencing themselves being young.

But the soul responds in a curious way, unlike the wife and children, or the employer and government who have been deceived through his wrong dealings. The soul responds by creating a pin which pricks his conscience, and this gnawing, antagonistic force within him he seeks to get rid of. He hides himself in jealousy, in the *sutala chakra*, until this becomes unacceptable. The confusion of the *talātala chakra* is no longer his pleasure. He can't hide there. So, he hides himself in anger and resentment—a cozy place within the *vitala chakra*—until this becomes unbearable. Then he hides himself in fear, in the *atala chakra*, fear of his own *purusha*, his own soul, his own psyche, his own seeing, until this becomes intolerable. Then he hides himself in memory and reason, and the being puts down its roots. The change in this individual can only be seen by the mellowness within his eyes and a new-born wisdom that is slowly developing in his conversations among those who knew him before.

Transmuting Willpower

Willpower is a *prāṇic* force which exudes out of the *maṇipūra chakra*. This energy, when directed downward, can be used up through excessive reason, excessive memorization, fear and amplification of fears, anger, the perpetuation of resentment without resolution, amplified by instinctive jealousies, all of which eventually dissipate the semi-divine energy of willpower and eventually close the *maṇipūra chakra*. But when this same energy of willpower is upwardly directed, it pulls memory into a purified memory, making it forget what has to be forgotten, namely wrong knowledge, and remember what has to be remembered—*siddhānta*, the final conclusions of the *ṛishis* who live within the *sahasrāra chakra,* the *siddhas* who are contacted through great *tapas.*

There is no reason to believe that developing and unfolding the ten petals of the *maṇipūra chakra* comes easily. To develop an indomitable will capable of the accomplishments needed as a prerequisite to make the upward climb to the *anāhata, viśuddha, ājñā* and *sahasrāra chakras,* and to sustain the benign attitudes of humility, is certainly not an easy task. But it comes naturally to one who has attained such in prior lifetimes, an older soul, I would say. Fulfilling each task one has begun, putting the cap back on the toothpaste tube after squeezing the toothpaste on the brush, the little things, and perfecting the *yamas* and the *niyamas,* especially contentment, austerity, giving, faith and regular worship, builds this indomitable will. These are mini-*sādhanas* one can perform on his own without the guidance of a *guru.* Yes, it is the little things that build the indomitable will that dominates the external intellect, its memory and reason abilities, and the instinctive impulses of fear, anger and jealousy. Doing this is just becoming a good person.

Willpower is the muscle of the mind. We lift weights, exercise, run a mile, all to develop the muscles of the physical body. The more we perform these practices, the more muscular we become. The process of strain reshapes the cellular properties and the structure of the muscles. Intermittent rest allows them to build up double. Strong muscles appear on the body as a result. The *maṇipūra chakra* is the sun center of the physical body and of the astral body, the place where all nerve currents of these two bodies meet and merge. It emanates the power of life. It is the seat of fire, the *agni homa.* It is the bridge between the ultimate illumination and a prolonged, ongoing, intellectual processing of ideas, coupled with instinctive willfulness. Let there be no mistake, we must get beyond that by transmuting this tool, willpower, into *mati,* cognition, where its energies are usable yet benign. Therefore, the more you use your personal, individual willpower in your religious service, in your business life, your personal life, your home life, your temple life, in fulfilling all the *yamas* and *niyamas,* the more willpower you have. It is an accumulative, ever-growing bank account.

Of course, you can lose some of it through lapses into fear, anger and jealousy, just as in an economic depression one loses money. But you can also court an inflation by seeking higher consciousness in the *viśuddha chakra* of divine love through the *anāhata chakra* of direct cognition, through understanding the oneness of a well-ordered, just universe, both inner and outer.

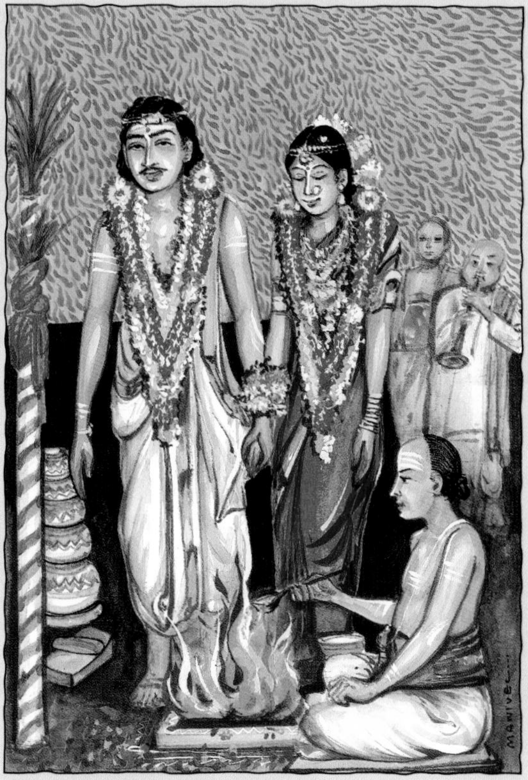

A couple voice their wedding vows, vrata, *promising life-long fidelity in one of our most sacred rites of passage.*

❁

Summary of the Eighth Observance

Embrace religious vows, rules and observances and never waver in fulfilling them. Honor vows as spiritual contracts with your soul, your community, with God, Gods and *guru.* Take vows to harness the instinctive nature. Fast periodically. Pilgrimage yearly. Uphold your vows strictly, be they chastity, marriage, monasticism, nonaddiction, tithing, loyalty to a lineage, vegetarianism or nonsmoking.

THE EIGHTH OBSERVANCE

Sacred Vows

Vrata व्रत

V*RATA*, TAKING SACRED VOWS, IS THE EIGHTH *NIYAMA* AND SOMETHING EVERY HINDU MUST DO AT ONE TIME OR ANOTHER DURING HIS LIFETIME. THE *BRAHMACHARYA VRATA* is the first, pledging to maintain virginity until marriage. The *vivāha vrata,* marriage vows, would generally be the next. Taking a vow is a sacred trust between yourself, your outer self, your inner self, your loved ones and closest friends. Even though they may not know of the vow you may have taken, it would be difficult to look them straight in the eye if you yourself know you have let yourself down. A vow is a sacred trust between you and your guardian *devas,* the *devas* that surround the temple you most frequent and the Mahādevas, who live within the Third World—which you live in, too, in your deep, innermost mind, in the radiant, self-luminous body of your soul.

Many people make little promises and break them. This is not a *vrata,* a sacred trust. A *vrata* is a sacred trust with God, Gods and *guru* made at a most auspicious time in one's life. *Vrata* is a binding force, binding the external mind to the soul and the soul to the Divine, though *vrata* is sometimes defined generally as following religious virtues or observances, following the principles of the *Vedas,* of the Hindu Dharma. There are *vratas* of many kinds, on many different levels, from the simple promise we make to ourself and our religious community and *guru* to perform the basic spiritual obligations, to the most specific religious vows.

Vratas give the strength to withstand the temptations of the instinctive forces that naturally come up as one goes on through life—not to suppress them but to rechannel them into a lifestyle fully in accord with the *yamas* and *niyamas*. The *yamas* should be at least two-thirds perfected and the *niyamas* two-thirds in effect before *vratas* are taken.

We must remember that the *yamas* are restraints, ten clues as to what forces to restrain and how to restrain them. Some people are better than others at accomplishing this, depending on their *prārabdha karmas,* but the effort in trying is the important thing. The practices, *niyamas,* on the other hand, are progressive, according to the perfection of the restraints. Commitment to the first *yama,* noninjury, *ahiṁsā,* for example, makes the first *niyama,* remorse, or *hrī,* a possibility in one's life. And *satya,* truthfulness, brings *santosha*—contentment, joy and serenity in life. The first five practices, *niyamas,* are tools to keep working with yourself, to keep trying within the five major areas they outline.

If one wants to progress further, he does not have to take on a *guru*—to study scriptures or develop a spiritual will or intellect—that would come naturally, nor to take simple *vratas,* to chant *Aum* as *japa* and to perform certain *sādhanas* and penance. These are all available. But a *guru* naturally comes into one's life when the last five *yamas*—steadfastness, compassion, honesty, a moderate appetite, and purity—give rise to the last five *niyamas*—*siddhānta śravaṇa* (choice of lineage), *mati* (cognition and developing a spiritual will with the *guru's* guidance), *vrata* (sacred vows before a *guru*), *japa* (recitation after initiation from *guru*) and *tapas* (austerities performed under the careful guidance of a *guru*). We can see that the last five practices are taken on two levels: *guru* involvement, and community and personal involvement.

Types of Vows

Many people get together with modern-day *gurus* and want to rush ahead, and with feigned humility seek to "get on with it" and "be their own person," but feel they need an initiation to do so. The *gurus* and *swāmīs* from India following a traditional path put initiation before them. Most *gurus* and *swāmīs* are dumbfounded by the devotion they see in these souls, perhaps not realizing they are stimulated by drugs and the desire to get something without earning it. The *gurus* presume they are already performing the *yamas* and *niyamas* and have dropped out of some higher inner world into Earth bodies. So, the initiations are given and vows are taken, but then when the reaction to the action comes within the mind of the devotee, and the *swāmī* begins to teach on a different level to this chosen group, because after initiation a new form of teaching and dissemination of inner knowledge occurs, and since it was only the initiation that was sought for (and he or she does not believe in God and the Gods and is not even part of the Hindu religion), once the devotee feels the pressure of responsibility, he or she responds by leaving, and even defaming the *guru*.

Many people think that initiation is like a graduation, the end of study. This is not true. Initiation is the beginning of study, the beginning of *sādhana*, the beginning of learning. Therefore, think well before you become initiated, because your loyalty is expected, and you are expected to adhere to the teachings of the *sampradāya*, of the lineage, into which you are initiated. This does not mean you can't attend temples or other religious activities of other *sampradāyas* occasionally, such as festivals, or listen to music or chants of other traditions occasionally, but this should be minimized so that your focus and concentration is upon what you were initiated into, because you are expected to advance on the path of that particular lineage.

There are certain simple vows in Hinduism which are easy to take and often are taken, such as, "If I'm successful in this business dealing, I will give twenty percent of the profits to my temple." Or, "If my spouse comes back to me, I shall always obey the *strī dharma* principles (or *purusha dharma*), be dedicated and devoted always." "If my dear mother, who is so devoted to my children, lives through her cancer operation (and Lord Gaṇeśa, the doctors have said the chances are not good), you will see me at the temple every Friday without fail. This is my *vrata*, Lord Gaṇeśa, and I say no more." We take vows to change our ways, vows to meditate daily, vows to desist from lying, vows to not eat meat, vows to remain celibate, vows to obey the *guru* and his tradition, vows to follow these *yamas* and *niyamas*.

Perhaps the most obvious and important vow, which can be taken most readily and renewed once a year on a day which you consider your most sacred day—such as Śivarātri, Gaṇeśa Chatūrthi, Skanda Shashṭhī or Dīpāvalī—is the *yama* and *niyama vrata*. These twenty restraints and practices are easy to memorize. Commit them to memory. The *vrata* should go like this: "O Lord Gaṇeśa, open the portals of my wisdom that I might take this *vrata* with open heart and clear mind. O Lord Murugan, give me the will, fortitude and renewed strength every step of the way to fulfill the *vrata* that I am taking. O Lord Śiva, forgive me if I fail, for these twenty restraints and practices are truly beyond my ability to perfectly uphold. So, this first year, Lord Śiva, I vow to fulfill these lofty ideals, to the best of my ability, at least fifty percent. I know I am weak. You know I am weak. I know you will make me strong. I know that you are drawing me ever patiently toward your holy feet. But, Lord Śiva, next year I will faithfully renew this *vrata*, this sacred vow, to these rules, these observances. And if I have succeeded in fulfilling my meager fifty percent according to my conscience, that shall increase my dedication and devotion to you, Lord Śiva, and I shall determine to fulfill the *yamas* and *niyamas* in my life and soul seventy-five percent or more."

Success and Failure

Many people feel that when they don't fulfill their *vrata* they have failed. One practical example to the contrary is Mahatma Gandhi, who took a vow to be celibate but broke it many times, yet continued the effort and ultimately conquered his instinctive nature. In taking a *vrata,* at the moment it is heard by priests, elders and all community members, when one hears oneself taking it, and all three worlds rejoice, a balanced scale has been created. Success is on one side, failure on the other. One or the other will win out. This is where the unreserved worship of Lord Murugan will help overbalance the scale on the success side. But if the scale teeters and wavers, the blessings and knowledge of the elders of the community should be sought: the mothers and fathers, the old aunties and uncles, the priests, the *pandits* and sages, the *ṛishis* and *gurus.* This and this alone will steady the balance. But if actual failure occurs, Lord Gaṇeśa Himself will catch the fall in His four arms and trunk. He will hold the devotee from going into the abyss of remorse of the darkness of the lower worlds. He will speak softly into the right ear and encourage that the *vrata* be immediately renewed, lest time elapse and the *asura* of depression take over mind, body and emotion. Yes, the only failure is that experienced by the one who quits, gives up, turns his back on the path and walks the other way, into the realms of darkness, beyond even the reach of the Gods. As Tiruvalluvar said, it is better to strive to fulfill great aspirations, even if you fail, than to achieve minor goals in life. Yes, this is very true.

On the everyday level there are *vratas* or contracts made with people of the outside world whom you don't even know. Buy a piece of property, and once you sign the contract you are bound to fulfill it. But a religious *vrata* is a contract between yourself, the religious community, the *devas* and the Gods and your *guru,* if you have one, all of whom know that human failure is a part of life; but striving is the fulfillment of life, and practice is the strengthening effect that the exercise of the human and spiritual will have over the baser elements.

Vows before the community, such as those of marriage and celibacy and other vows where community support is needed, are very important. Other, more personal vows are taken before the community, a temple priest, *pandit,* elder, *swāmī, guru,* or *satguru* if help is needed to strengthen the individual's ability to fulfill them. For a certain type of person, a vow before Lord Gaṇeśa, Lord Murugan, Lord Śiva or all three is enough for him to gain strength and fulfill it. A vow is never only to oneself. This is important to remember. A vow is always to God, Gods and *guru,* community and respected elders.

One cannot make one's vow privately, to one's own individual *āṇava,* external personal ego, thinking that no one is listening. This would be more of a promise to oneself, like a New Year's resolution, a change in attitude based on a new belief, all of which has nothing to do with the *yamas* and *niyamas* or religion.

In speaking about the *yama* and *niyama vrata,* there is no difference in how the family person upholds it and the celibate monastic upholds it. The families are in their home, the monks are in their *maṭha,* monastery. In regards to the *vrata* of sexual purity, for example, the family man vows to be faithful to his wife and to treat all other women as either a mother or sister and to have no sexual thoughts, feelings or fantasies toward them. *Sadhākas, yogīs* and *swāmīs* vow to look at all women as their mothers or sisters, and God Śiva and their *guru* as their mother and father. There is no difference.

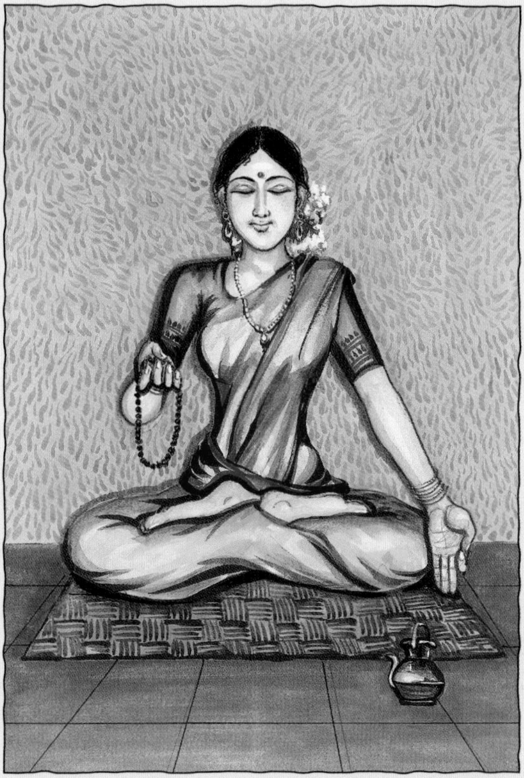

A Hindu woman chants her mantra *on a* mālā *of holy beads, performing* japa *during her morning* sādhana.

Summary of the Ninth Observance

Chant your holy *mantra* daily, reciting the sacred sound, word or phrase given by your *guru.* Bathe first, quiet the mind and concentrate fully to let *japa* harmonize, purify and uplift you. Heed your instructions and chant the prescribed repetitions without fail. Live free of anger so that *japa* strengthens your higher nature. Let *japa* quell emotions and quiet the rivers of thought.

THE NINTH OBSERVANCE

Recitation

Japa जप

NOW WE SHALL FOCUS ON *JAPA*, RECITATION OF HOLY *MANTRAS*, THE NINTH *NIYAMA*. HERE AGAIN, A *GURU* IS ESSENTIAL, UNLESS ONLY THE SIMPLEST OF MANTRAS ARE RECITED. The simplest of *mantras* is Aum, pronounced "AA, OO, MMM." The AA balances the physical forces when pronounced separately from the OO and the MMM, as the OO balances the astral and mental bodies. The MMM brings the spiritual body into the foreground. And when pronounced all together, AA-OO-MMM, all three bodies are harmonized. *Aum* is a safe *mantra* which may be performed without a *guru's* guidance by anyone of any religious background living on this planet, as it is the primal sound of the universe itself. All sounds blended together make the sound "Aum." The overtone of the sounds of an entire city would be "Aum." In short, it harmonizes, purifies and uplifts the devotee.

One might ask why a *guru* is important to perform such a simple task as *japa*. It is the *śakti* of the *guru*, of the Gods and the *devas* that give power to the *mantra*. Two people, a civilian and a policeman, could say to a third person, "Stop in the name of the law." The third person would only obey one of them. The one who had no authority would not be listened to. In this example, the policeman had been initiated and had full authority. Therefore, his *mantra*, "Stop in the name of the law," seven words, had the desired effect. The person who had not been initiated said the same words, but nobody paid any attention to him. Now, this does not mean one can choose a *guru*, study with the *guru*, become accepted by the *guru*, feign humility, do all the right things and say all the right words, become initiated, receive the *mantra* and then be off into some kind of other activities or opt for a more liberal path. The *guru's* disdain would diminish if not cancel the benefits of the initiation, which obviously had been deceptively achieved. This is why *siddhānta śravana* (choosing your path carefully) and *mati* (choosing your *guru* carefully, being loyal to the *sampradāya,* to your *guru* and his successor or successors and training your children to be loyal to the *sampradāya)* are the foundation of character that the first fifteen restraints and practices are supposed to produce.

Mantra initiation is *guru dīkshā.* Traditionally, the family *guru* would give *mantra dīkshā* to the mother and the father and then to the young people, making the *guru* part of the family itself. There is no way that *mantras* can be sold and be effective. There is no way that the *dīkshā* of *mantra* initiation, which permits *japa,* could be effective for someone who was not striving to fulfill the first seventeen of the *yamas* and *niyamas.* Any wise *guru* would test the devotee on these before granting initiation. There is no way a *mantra* can be learned from a book and be effective. Therefore, approach the *guru* cautiously and with a full heart. When asked if you are restraining yourself according to the ten *yamas,* know that perfection is not expected, but effort is. And if you are practicing the first seven *niyamas,* know that perfection is not expected here either, but regular attentiveness to them is. You, the *guru,* your family and your friends will all know when you are on the threshold of *mantra dīkshā,* which when performed by an established *guru* is called *guru dīkshā.*

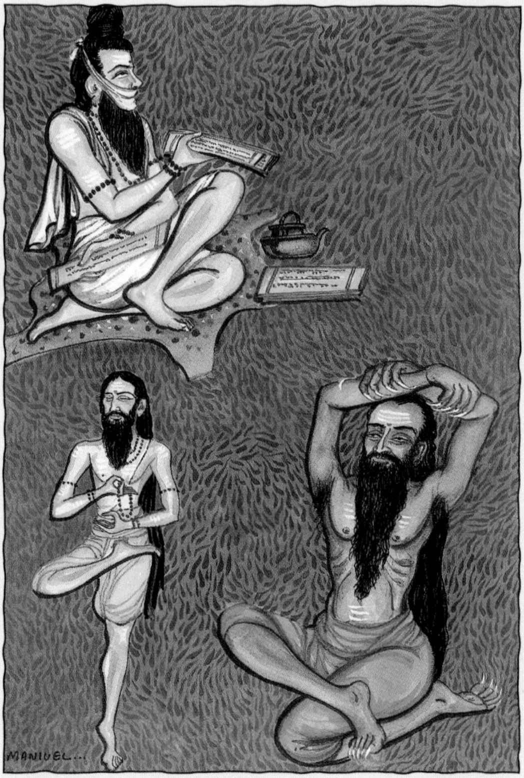

Religious austerity, tapas, *ranges from simple self-denial to rigorous* yogic *ordeals and physical challenges.*

Summary of the Tenth Observance

Practice austerity, serious disciplines, penance and sacrifice. Be ardent in worship, meditation and pilgrimage. Atone for misdeeds through penance *(prāyaśchitta),* such as 108 prostrations or fasting. Perform self-denial, giving up cherished possessions, money or time. Fulfill severe austerities at special times, under a *satguru's* guidance, to ignite the inner fires of self-transformation.

THE TENTH OBSERVANCE

Austerity & Sacrifice

Tapas तपस्

THE TENTH AND FINAL *NIYAMA* IS AUSTERITY, PERFORMING *SĀDHANA,* PENANCE, *TAPAS* AND SACRIFICE. ALL RELIGIONS OF THE WORLD HAVE THEIR FORMS OF AUSTERITY, conditions which one has to live up to—or which individuals are unable to live up to who are too lazy or too dull-minded to understand; and Hinduism is no exception. Our austerities start within the home in the form of daily *sādhana.* This is obligatory and includes *pūjā,* scriptural reading and chanting of holy *mantras.* This personal vigil takes about half an hour or more. Other *sādhanas* include pilgrimage to a far-off sacred place once a year, visiting a temple once a week, preferably on Friday or Monday, attending festivals and fulfilling *saṁskāras,* rites of passage, for the children especially, but all the family members as well. To atone for misdeeds, penance is obligatory. We must quickly mitigate future effects of the causes we have set into action. This is done through such acts as performing 108 prostrations before the God in the temple.

Tapas is even more austere. It may come early in a lifetime or later in life, unbidden or provoked by *rāja yoga* practices. It is the fire that straightens the twisted life and mind of an individual, bringing him into pure being, giving a new start in life, awakening higher consciousness and a cosmic relationship with God and the Gods, friends, relatives and casual acquaintances. *Tapas* in Hinduism is sought for, feared, suffered through and loved. Its pain is greater than the pains of parturition, but in the aftermath is quickly forgotten, as the soul, in childlike purity, shines forth in the joys of rebirth that follow in the new life.

Tapas is walking through fire, being scorched, burnt to a crisp, crawling out the other side unburnt, without scars, with no pain. *Tapas* is walking through the rain, completely drenched, and when the storm stops, not being wet. *Tapas* is living in a hurricane, tossed about on a churning ocean in a small boat, and when the storm subsides, being landed on a peaceful beach unharmed but purified. *Tapas* is a mind in turmoil, insane unto its very self. A psychic surgery is being performed by the Gods themselves. When the operation is over, the patient has been cut loose of the dross of all past lives. *Tapas* is a landslide of mud, a psychic earthquake, coming upon the head and consuming the body of its victim, smothering him in the dross of his misdeeds, beneath which he is unable to breathe, see, speak or hear. He awakens from this hideous dream resting on a mat in a garden hut, smelling sweet jasmine, seeing pictures of Gods and *devas* adorning the mud walls and hearing the sound of a flute coming from a distant source.

Truly, *tapas* in its fullest form is sought for only by the renunciate under the guidance of a *satguru*, but this madness often comes unbidden to anyone on this planet whose dross of misdeeds spills over. The only difference for the Hindu is that he knows what is happening and how it is to be handled; or at least the *gurus* know, the *swāmīs* know, the elders know, the astrologers know. This knowledge is built into the Hindu mind flow as grout is built into a stone wall.

A Lesson in Sacrifice

Sacrifice may be the least-practiced austerity, and the most important. It is the act of giving up to a greater power a cherished possession (be it money, time, intelligence or a physical object) to manifest a greater good. There are many ways to teach sacrifice. My *satguru* taught sacrifice by cooking a great feast for several hundred people, which took all day to prepare. Their mouths were watering. They had not eaten all day, so as to prepare their bodies to receive this *prasāda* from the *satguru*. The meal was scheduled to be served at high noon. But Satguru Yogaswami kept delaying, saying, "We have not yet reached the auspicious moment. Let us sing some more *bhajanas* and *Natchintanai*. Be patient." At about 3PM, he said, "Before we can partake of our *prasāda*, I shall ask eleven strong men here to dig a deep, square hole in the ground." They stepped forward and he indicated the spot where they should dig. Shovels were obtained from homes nearby, and the digging commenced. All waited patiently for his will to be fulfilled, the stomachs growling, the mouths watering at the luscious fragrances of the hot curries, the rasam and the freshly-boiled rice, five sweet-smelling curries, mango chutneys, dal, yogurt and delicious sweet *payasam*. It was a real feast.

Finally, just before dusk, the pit was completed, and the great saint indicated that it was time to serve the food. "Come, children, surround this pit," he said. Two or three hundred people stepped forward and surrounded the ten- by ten-foot hole. Women and children were sitting in the front and the men standing in the back, all wondering what he was going to say and hoping he would not delay any longer with the feast. He said, "Now we shall serve our *prasāda*." He called forward two of the huskiest of the eleven men, the strongest and biggest, and commanded, "Serve the rice. Bring the entire pot." It was a huge brass pot containing nearly 400 pounds of rice. By this time, many had left, as they had been cooking all morning and singing all afternoon. Only the most devout had remained to see the outcome. When the day began, 1,000 had come. The preparations were for a very big crowd.

Now he said, "Pour the rice in the middle of the pit." Banana leaves had been laid carefully at the bottom of the pit to form a giant serving plate. The crowd was aghast. "Pour it into the pit?" "Don't hesitate," he commanded. Though stunned, the men obeyed Yogaswami without question, dropping the huge mass of steaming rice onto the middle of the banana leaves. He told one man, "Bring the eggplant curry!" To another he said, "Go get the potato curry! We must make this a full and auspicious offering."

As all the curries were neatly placed around the rice, everyone was wondering, "Are we to all eat together out of the pit? Is this what the *guru* has in mind?" Then the *kulambu* sauce was poured over the middle of the rice. Five pounds of salt was added on the side. Sweet mango and ginger chutneys were placed in the proper way. One by one, each of the luscious preparations was placed in the pit, much to the dismay of those gathered.

Giving Back to Mother Earth

After all the food had been served, the *satguru* stood up and declared, "People, all of you, participate. Come forward." They immediately thought, finishing his sentence in their minds, "to eat together this luscious meal you have been waiting for all day as a family of *śishyas*." But he had something else in mind, and directed, "Pick up the eleven shovels, shovel some dirt over this delicious meal and then pass your shovel on to the next person. We have fed our Mother Earth, who has given so generously of her abundance all these many years to this large Śaivite community. Now we are sacrificing our *prasāda* as a precious, heartfelt gift. Mother Earth is hungry. She gets little back; we take all. Let this be a symbol to the world and to each of us that we must sacrifice what we want most."

In this way, our *satguru*, Śiva Yogaswami, began the first Earth worship ceremony in northern Sri Lanka. He taught a lesson of *tapas* and sacrifice, of fasting and giving, and giving and fasting. By now the hour was late, very late. After touching his feet and receiving the mark of Śiva from him in the form of *vibhūti,* holy ash, on their forehead, the devotees returned to their homes. It was too late to cook a hot meal, lest the neighbors smell the smoke and know that mischief was afoot. We are sure that a few, if not many, satisfied themselves with a few ripe bananas, while pondering the singular lesson the *satguru* had taught.

Let's worship the Earth. It is a being—intelligent and always giving. Our physical bodies are sustained by her abundance. When her abundance is withdrawn, our physical bodies are no more. The ecology of this planet is an intricate intelligence. Through sacrifice, which results in *tapas* and *sādhana,* we nurture Mother Earth's goodwill, friendliness and sustenance. Instill in yourself appreciation, recognition. We should not take advantage of all of this generosity, as a predator does of those he preys upon.

Yes, austerities are a vital part of all sects of Hinduism. They are a call of the soul to bring the outer person into the perfection that the soul is now, has always been and will always be. Austerities should be assigned by a *guru,* a *swāmī* or a qualified elder of the community. One should submit to wise guidance, because these *sādhanas,* penances, *tapas* and sacrifices lift our consciousness so that we can deal with, learn to live with, the perfection of the self-luminous, radiant, eternal being of the soul within. Austerity is the powerful bath of fire and bright rays of showering light that washes the soul clean of the dross of its many past lives, and of the current life, which have held it in the bondage of ignorance, misgiving, unforgivingness and the self-perpetuating ignorance of the truths of the Sanātana Dharma. "As the intense fire of the furnace refines gold to brilliance, so does the burning suffering of austerity purify the soul to resplendence" (*Weaver's Wisdom/Tirukural,* 267).

Conclusion

Samāpanam समापनम्

WE HAVE EXPLORED TOGETHER GURUDEVA'S ELUCIDATION OF THE TWENTY ANCIENT VEDIC TOOLS FOR SELF-TRANSFORMATION, PRACTICED THROUGH THE MILLENNIA BY tens of millions of seekers. Their challenges back then are no different than ours in modern times. It is always challenging to undertake the work of changing our habits, changing our thoughts, changing our attitudes, reactions and modes of action. Challenging, yet enormously rewarding when our efforts bear fruit.

Success in fulfilling the *yamas* and *niyamas* provides the stability in our life that sustained success in meditation requires. Without this stability, the ups and downs of life are paramount, and significant advancement in our spiritual life does not manifest. A tall building needs a solid foundation to sustain an earthquake without toppling. So, too, higher states of consciousness need the positive habits of the *yamas* and *niyamas* to be sustained through the challenges that inevitably come to us in life. The modern exponent of *haṭha yoga* B.K.S. Iyengar cautioned, "Practice of *āsanas* without the backing of *yama* and *niyama* is mere acrobatics. *Yama* and *niyama* control the *yogī's* passions and emotions and keep him in harmony with his fellow man." Sri Sri Anandamurthi taught, "In ancient times an aspirant had to practice *yamas* and *niyamas* for twelve years before he was even initiated. Without them, *sādhana* is an impossibility." Yogacharya Krpalvanand called *yama* and *niyama* the "impenetrable fort of *yoga*," and he warned, "If they are neglected, many hurdles crop up during *sādhana*, and it takes a very long time to uproot those evils."

One of the misconceptions you may have intuited as you studied these lessons is that we can take refuge in the higher practices of the *niyamas* and avoid the more difficult work of the *yamas*. This is a misconception widely held, and perfectly flawed. We must stay focused on the difficult work of the *yamas* at the outset, make commitments to harness our instinctive nature, our desires, our lazy patterns of life. Only then can the life energies flow freely into the *niyamas*, bringing the positive spiritual practices into their maturity.

Gurudeva has given us a great map of the mind in his interpretations of the *yamas* and *niyamas*. Nowhere else will you find his pairing of the one with the other, of each *yama* with a specific *niyama*. He knew, from the deepest part of human knowing, that the positive and the negative are intertwined, that the resolution of the lower nature allows for the natural expression of the higher, just as a balloon suddenly soars skyward when it drops off its sandbags.

So, as you carry on in the work ahead, on the path ahead, as you work with the *yamas* and *niyamas* in your life, don't settle for the easy path of worshiping unless you have dealt with the harder path of mastering patience; don't be content with your progress in contentment until you are truly truthful in all your dealings with others; don't be satisfied with your charitibleness until even the thought of stealing has been eliminated from your heart; don't practice *japa* in earnest unless you have become a vegetarian; don't pursue serious austerities without a good foundation in purity.

As Gurudeva wrote in *Dancing with Śiva*, "Good conduct is a combination of avoiding unethical behavior and performing virtuous, spiritualizing acts." Now you have the pattern, in Hinduism's code of conduct. Proceed with confidence.

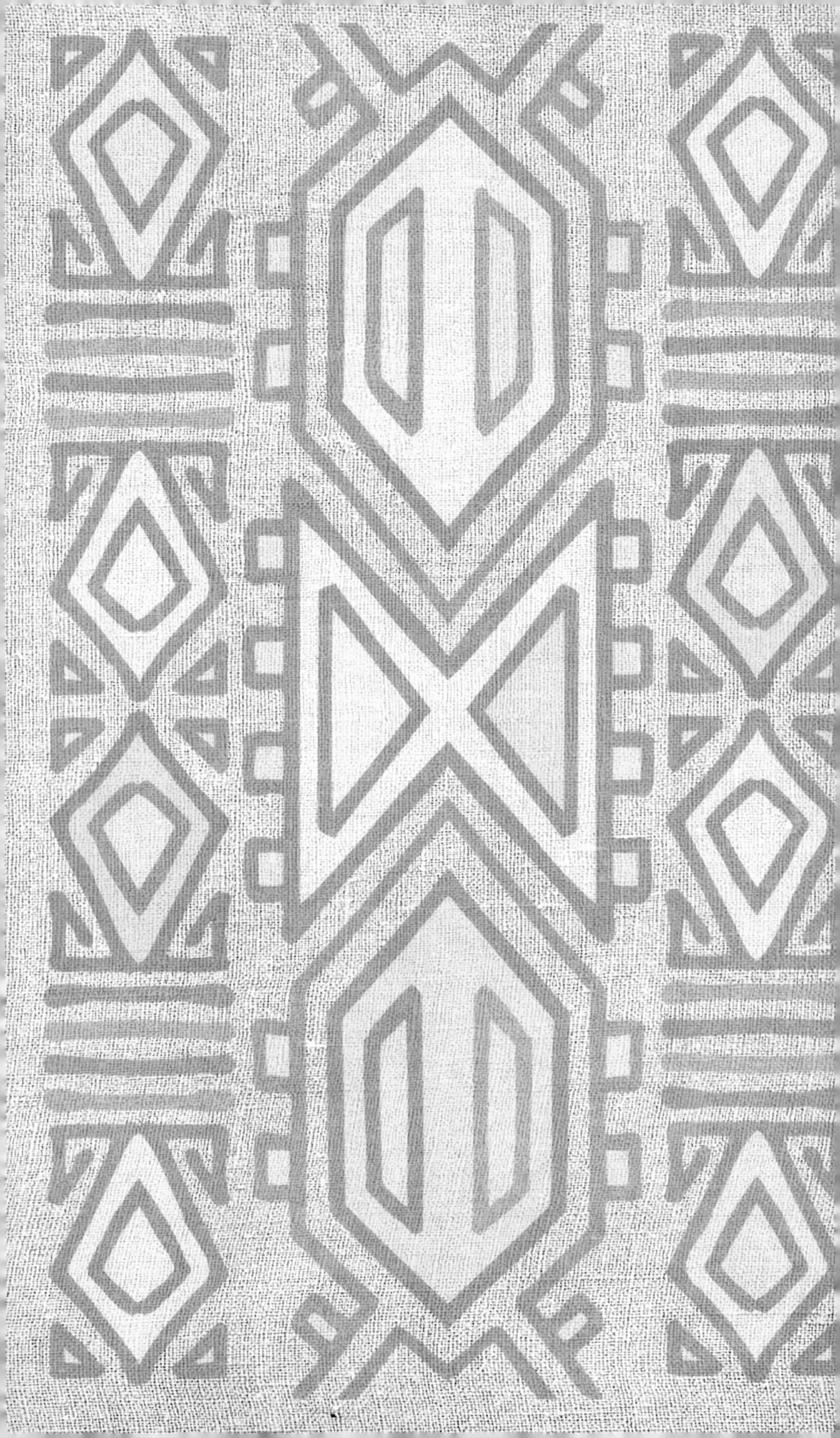

Glossary

Śabda Kośaḥ शब्दकोशः

aadheenam: ஆதீனம் A Śaivite Hindu monastery and temple complex in the South Indian Śaiva Siddhānta tradition. The *aadheenam* head is called the *guru mahāsannidhānam* or *aadheenakarthar.*

Absolute: Lower case (absolute): real, not dependent on anything else, not relative. Upper case (Absolute): Ultimate Reality, the unmanifest, unchanging and transcendent Paraśiva. See: *Paraśiva.*

āchārya: आचार्य A highly respected teacher.

actinic: Spiritual, creating light. Adjective derived from the Greek *aktis,* "ray." Of or pertaining to consciousness in its pure, unadulterated state. Actinic force is the superconscious mind and not a force which comes from the superconcious mind. Commonly known as life, spirit, it can be seen as the light in man's eyes; it is the force that leaves man when he leaves his odic physical body behind. It is not opposite to odic force, it is different than odic force as light is different than water but shines through it. Actinic force flows freely through odic force. See: *kośa.*

advaita: अद्वैत "Non-dual; not twofold." Nonduality or monism. The doctrine that Ultimate Reality consists of a one principle substance, or God. Opposite of *dvaita,* dualism. See: *dvaita-advaita, Vedānta.*

Advaita Īśvaravāda: अद्वैत ईश्वरवाद "Nondual and Personal-God-as-Ruler doctrine," *monistic theism.* The philosophy of the *Vedas* and *Śaiva Āgamas,* which believes in the ultimate oneness of all things and in the reality of the personal Deity.

Advaita Īśvaravādin: अद्वैत ईश्वरवादिन् A follower of Advaita Īśvaravāda.

Advaita Siddhānta: अद्वैत सिद्धान्त "Nondual perfect conclusions." Śaivite philosophy codified in the *Āgamas* which has at its core the nondual (*advaitic*) identity of God, soul and world. with a strong emphasis on internal and external worship, *yoga sādhanas* and *tapas. Advaita Siddhānta* is a term used in South India to distinguish Tirumular's school from the pluralistic Siddhānta of Meykandar and Aghorasiva. It is the philosophy of this contemporary Hindu catechism.

Āgama: आगम The tradition that which has "come down." An enormous collection of Sanskrit scriptures which, along with the *Vedas,* are revered as *śruti* (revealed scripture). The primary source and authority for ritual, *yoga* and temple construction.

agni: अग्नि "Fire." 1) One of the five elements, *pañchabhūta.* 2) God of the element fire, invoked through Vedic ritual known as *yajña, agnikāraka, homa* and *havana;* the divine messenger who receives prayers and oblations and conveys them to the heavenly spheres. See: *yajña.*

ahiṁsā: अहिंसा "Noninjury," nonviolence or nonhurtfulness. Not causing harm to others, physically, mentally or emotionally. See: *yama-niyama.*

ājñā chakra: आज्ञाचक्र "Command wheel." The third-eye center. See: *chakra.*

ākāśa: आकाश "Space." The sky. Free, open space. Ether, the fifth and most subtle of the five elements—earth, air, fire, water and ether. Empirically, the rarefied space or ethereal fluid plasma that pervades the universes, inner and outer. Esoterically, mind, the superconscious strata holding all that exists and all that potentially exists, wherein all happenings are recorded and can be read by clairvoyants.

all-pervasive: Diffused throughout or existing in every part of the universe.

anāhata chakra: **अनाहतचक्र** "Wheel of unstruck [sound]." The heart center. See: *chakra.*

ānanda: **आनन्द्** "Bliss." The pure joy—ecstasy or enstasy—of God-consciousness or spiritual experience.

ānandamaya kośa: **आनन्दमयकोश** "Bliss body." The body of the soul, which ultimately merges with Śiva. See: *kośa, soul.*

āṇava mala: **आणवमल** "Impurity of smallness; finitizing principle." God's individualizing veil of duality that enshrouds the soul. It is the source of finitude and ignorance, the most basic of the three bonds *(āṇava, karma, māyā)* which temporarily limit the soul.

antyeshṭi: **अन्त्येष्टि** "Last rites." Funeral.

anugraha śakti: **अनुग्रहशक्ति** "Graceful or favoring power." Revealing grace. God Śiva's power of illumination, through which the soul is freed from the bonds of *āṇava, karma* and *māyā* and ultimately attains liberation, *moksha.* Specifically, *anugraha* descends on the soul as *śaktipāta,* the *dīkshā* (initiation) from a *satguru. Anugraha* is a key concept in Śaiva Siddhānta. It comes when *āṇava mala,* the shell of finitude which surrounds the soul, reaches a state of ripeness, *malaparipāka.* See: *grace, śaktinipāta.*

ārjava: **आर्जव** "Steadfastness." See: *yama-niyama.*

arul: **அருள்** "Grace." The third of the three stages of the *sakala avasthai* when the soul yearns for the grace of God, *śaktinipāta.* At this stage the soul seeks *pati-jñānam,* knowledge of God. See: *pati-jñānam, sakala avasthā, śaktinipāta.*

āsana: **आसन** "Seat; posture." In *haṭha yoga, āsana* refers to any of numerous poses prescribed to balance and tune up the subtle energies of mind and body for meditation and to promote health and longevity.

ashṭāṅga yoga: **अष्टाङ्गयोग** "Eight-limbed union." The classical *rāja yoga* system of eight progressive stagesto Illumination: 1) ***—yama:*** "Restraint." Virtuous and moral living 2) ***—niyama***: "Observance." Religious practices which cultivate the qualities of the higher nature. 3) ***—āsana:*** "Seat or posture." 4) ***—prāṇāyāma:*** "Mastering life force."Breath control. 5) ***—pratyāhāra:*** "Withdrawal." Withdrawing consciousness from the physical senses. 6) ***—dhāraṇā:*** "Concentration." Guiding the flow of consciousness. 7) ***—dhyāna:*** "Meditation." 8) ***—samādhi:*** "Enstasy," "sameness, contemplation/realization." See: *yoga.*

āśrama: **आश्रम** "Place of striving." Hermitage; order of the life. Holy sanctuary; the residence and teaching center of a *sādhu,* saint, *swāmī,* ascetic or *guru;* often includes lodging for students. Also names life's four stages.

asteya: **अस्तेय** "Nonstealing." See: *yama-niyama.*

āstikya: **आस्तिक्य** "Faith." See: *yama-niyama.*

astral body: The subtle, nonphysical body *(sūkshma śarīra)* in which the soul functions in the astral plane, the inner world also called Antarloka. See: *kośa, soul.*

astral plane (or world): The subtle world, or Antarloka, spanning the spectrum of consciousness from the *viśuddha chakra* in the throat to the *pātāla chakra* in the soles of the feet. In the astral plane, the soul is enshrouded in the astral body, called *sūkshma śarīra.* See: *astral body, loka, three worlds.*

asura: **असुर** "Evil spirit; demon." (Opposite of *sura: "deva;* God.") A being of the lower astral plane, Naraka. *Asuras* can and do interact with the physical plane, causing major and minor problems in people's lives. *Asuras* do evolve and do not remain permanently in this state.

atala chakra: अतल चक्र "Bottomless region." The first *chakra* below the *mūlādhāra,* at the hip level. Region of fear and lust. See: *chakra, Narakaloka.*

Aum: ॐ or ओम् Often spelled *Om.* The mystic syllable of Hinduism, associated with Lord Gaṇeśa, placed at the beginning of sacred writings. In common usage in several Indian languages, *aum* means "yes, verily" or "hail." See: *Praṇava.*

aura: The luminous colorful field of subtle energy radiating within and around the human body. The colors change according to the ebb and flow of one's state of consciousness, thoughts, moods and emotions.

avasthā: अवस्था (Tamil: *avasthai.*) "Condition or state" of consciousness or experience. 1) Any of three stages of the soul's evolution from the point of its creation to final merger in the Primal Soul. 2) The states of consciousness as discussed in the *Māṇḍūkya Upanishad: jāgrat* (or *vaiśvānara),* "wakefulness;" *svapna* (or *taijasa),* "dreaming;" *sushupti,* "deep sleep;" and *turīya,* "the fourth" state, of superconsciousness. A fifth state, "beyond *turīya,*" is *turīyātīta.* See: *kevala avasthā, sakala avasthā, śuddha avasthā.*

awareness: Individual consciousness, perception, knowing; the witness of perception, the "inner eye of the soul." *Sākshin* or *chit* in Sanskrit.

āyurveda: आयुर्वेद "Science of life." A holistic system of medicine and health native to ancient India, seeking *āyus,* "longevity," and *ārogya,* "diseaselessness," to facilitate spiritual progress. Focus is on balancing energies through methods suited to the individual's constitution, lifestyle and nature.

Ayyappan: ஐயப்பன் Popular God of a recently formed sect that focuses on pilgrimage to the top of Sabarimalai, a sacred hill in Kerala.

Being: When capitalized, *being* refers to God's essential divine nature—Pure Consciousness, Absolute Reality and Primal Soul (God's nature as a divine Person). Lower case *being* refers to the essential nature of a person, that within which never changes; existence. See: *Śiva.*

bhajana: भजन Spiritual song. Individual or group singing of devotional songs, hymns and chants.

bhūmikā: भूमिका "Earth; ground; soil." Preface; introduction to a book. From *bhū,* "to become, exist; arise, come into being."

Bodhinatha (Bodhinātha): बोधिनाथ "Lord of Wisdom." The current preceptor of the Nandinātha Sampradāya's Kailāsa Paramparā, and Guru Mahāsannidhānam of Kauai Aadheenam, ordained by Satguru, Sivaya Subramuniyaswami in 2001.

brahmachārī: ब्रह्मचारी An unmarried male spiritual aspirant who practices continence, observes religious disciplines, including *sādhana,* devotion and service and who may be under simple vows. Also names one in the student stage, age 12–24, or until marriage.

brahmachāriṇī: ब्रह्मचारिणी Feminine counterpart of *brahmachārī.*

brahmacharya: ब्रह्मचर्य See: *yama-niyama.*

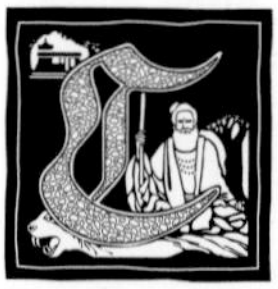

chakra: चक्र "Wheel." Any of the nerve plexes or centers of force and consciousness located within the *inner bodies* of man. In the physical body there are corresponding nerve plexuses, ganglia and glands. The seven principal *chakras* are situated along the spinal cord from the base to the cranial chamber. Additionally, seven *chakras* exist below the spine. They are seats of instinctive consciousness, the origin of jealousy, hatred, envy, guilt, sorrow, etc. They constitute the lower or hellish world, called *Naraka* or *pātāla.* Thus, there are 14 major *chakras* in all. The seven upper chakras are: 1) ***mūlādhāra*** (base of spine): memory, time and space; 2) ***svādhishṭhāna*** (below navel): reason; 3) ***maṇipūra*** (solar plexus): willpower; 4) ***anāhata*** (heart center): direct cognition; 5) ***viśuddha*** (throat): divine love; 6) ***ājñā*** (third eye): divine sight; 7) ***sahasrāra*** (crown of head): illumination, Godliness. The seven lower *chakras* are 1) ***atala*** (hips): fear and lust; 2) ***vitala*** (thighs): raging anger; 3) ***sutala*** (knees): retaliatory jealousy; 4) ***talātala*** (calves): prolonged mental confusion; 5) ***rasātala*** (ankles): selfishness; 6) ***mahātala*** (feet): absence of conscience; 7) ***pātāla*** (located in the soles of the feet): murder and malice. See: *Narakaloka.*

clairaudience: "Clear-hearing." Psychic or divine hearing, *divyaśravana.* The ability to hear the inner currents of the nervous system, the *Aum* and other mystic tones. Hearing in one's mind the words of inner-plane beings or earthly beings not physically present. Also, hearing the highe "eee" sound, or *nādanāḍī śakti,* through the day or while in meditation.

clairvoyance: "Clear-seeing." Psychic or divine sight, *divyadṛishṭi.* The ability to look into the inner worlds and see auras, *chakras, nāḍīs,* thought forms, non-physical people and subtle forces.

concentration: Uninterrupted and sustained attention. See: *ashṭaṅga yoga.*

conscious mind: The external, everyday state of consciousness. See: *mind.*

consciousness: *Chitta* or *chaitanya.* 1) A synonym for mind-stuff, *chitta;* or 2) the condition or power of perception, awareness, apprehension.

contemplation: Religious or mystical absorption beyond meditation.

cosmos: The universe, or whole of creation, especially with reference to its order, harmony and completeness. See: *loka, three worlds.*

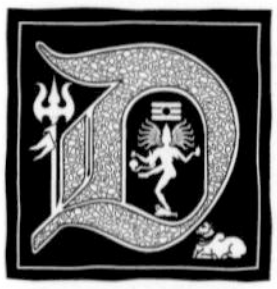

Dakshiṇāmūrti: दक्षिणामूर्ति "South-facing form." Lord Śiva depicted sitting under a banyan tree, silently teaching four *ṛishis* at His feet. See: *Śiva.*

dāna: दान Generosity, giving. See: *yama-niyama.*

daśama bhāga vrata: दशमभागव्रत "One-tenth-part vow." A promise that tithers make before God, Gods and their family or peers to tithe regularly.

daśamāṁśa: दशमांश "One-tenth sharing." The traditional Hindu practice of tithing, giving one-tenth of one's income to a religious institution.

dayā: दया "Compassion." See: *yama-niyama.*

Deity: "God." The image or *mūrti* installed in a temple or the Mahādeva the *mūrti* represents.

deva: देव "Shining one." A being inhabiting the higher astral plane, in a subtle, non-physical body. *Deva* is also used in scripture to mean "God or Deity."

Devaloka: देवलोक "Plane of radiant beings." A synonym of Maharloka, the higher astral plane, realm of *anāhata chakra.* See: *loka.*

devonic: Of or relating to the *devas* or their world.

dhāraṇā: धारणा "Concentration." From *dhṛi,* "to hold." See: *ashṭaṅga yoga.*

dharma: धर्म From *dhṛi,* "to sustain; carry, hold." Hence *dharma* is "that which contains or upholds the cosmos." *Dharma* has manifold meanings, including: divine law, ethics, law of being, way of righteousness, religion, duty, virtue, justice, goodness and truth. Essentially, *dharma* is the orderly fulfillment of an inherent nature or destiny. Relating to the soul, it is the mode of conduct most conducive to spiritual advancement, the right and righteous path. There are four principal kinds of *dharma,* known collectively as ***chaturdharma:*** "four religious laws." 1) ***ṛita:*** "Universal law." The laws of being and nature that contain and govern all forms, functions and processes, from galaxy clusters to the power of mental thought and perception. 2) ***varṇa dharma***: "Law of one's kind." Social duty. *Varṇa* can mean "race, tribe, appearance, character, color, social standing, etc." Obligations and responsibilities within one's nation, society, community, class, occupational subgroup and family. 3) ***āśrama dharma:*** "Duties of life's stages." Human or developmental *dharma,* fulfilling of the duties of the four stages of life—*brahmachārī* (student), *gṛihastha* (householder), *vānaprastha* (elder advisor) and *sannyāsa* (religious solitaire). 4) ***svadharma***: "Personal obligations or duty." One's perfect individual pattern through life, according to one's own particular physical, mental and emotional nature, the application of *dharma,* dependent on personal *karma,* reflected in one's race, community, physical characteristics, health, intelligence, skills and aptitudes, desires and tendencies, religion, *sampradāya,* family and *guru.*

dhṛiti: धृति "Steadfastness." See: *yama-niyama.*

dhyāna: ध्यान "Meditation." See: *ashṭaṅga yoga.*

dīkshā: दीक्षा "Initiation." Solemn induction by which one is entered into a new realm of spiritual awareness and practice by a teacher or preceptor through bestowing of blessings. Denotes initial or deepened connection with the teacher and his lineage and is usually accompanied by ceremony.

Dīpāvalī: दीपावली "Row of Lights." A very popular home and community festival in October/November when Hindus of all denominations light oil or electric lights and set off fireworks in a joyful celebration of the victory of good over evil and light over darkness.

disincarnate: Having no physical body; of the astral plane; astral beings. See: *astral body, astral plane.*

dvaita-advaita: द्वैत अद्वैत "Dual-nondual; twoness-not twoness." Among the most important categories in the classification of Hindu philosophies. *Dvaita* and *advaita* define two ends of a vast spectrum. —***dvaita:*** The doctrine of dualism, according to which reality is ultimately composed of two irreducible principles, entities, truths, etc. God and soul, for example, are seen as eternally separate. —**dualistic:** Of or relating to dualism, concepts, writings, theories which treat dualities (good-and-evil, high-and-low, them-and-us) as fixed, rather than transcendable. —**pluralism:** A form of nonmonism which emphasizes three or more eternally separate realities, e.g., God, soul and world. —***advaita:*** The doctrine of nondualism or monism, that reality is ultimately composed of one whole principle, substance or God, with no independent parts. In essence, all is God. —**monistic theism:** A dipolar view which encompasses both monism and dualism.

dualism: See: *dvaita-advaita.*

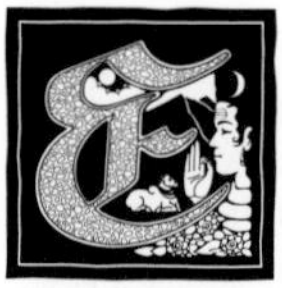

ego: The external personality or sense of "I" and "mine." Broadly, individual identity. In Śaiva Siddhānta and other schools, the ego is equated with the *tattva* of *ahaṁkāra,* "I-maker," which bestows the sense of I-ness, individuality and separateness from God.

eminent: High; above others in stature, rank or achievement.

enlightenment: For Śaiva monists, Self Realization, *samādhi* without seed *(nirvikalpa samādhi);* the ultimate attainment, sometimes referred to as Paramātma *darśana,* or as *ātma darśana,* "Self vision."

existentialism: A philosophy that emphasizes the uniqueness and isolation of the individual experience in a hostile or indifferent universe, regards human existence as unexplainable, and stresses freedom of choice and responsibility for the consequences of one's acts.

existentialist: Pertaining to, or believing in, the philosophy of *existentialism.*

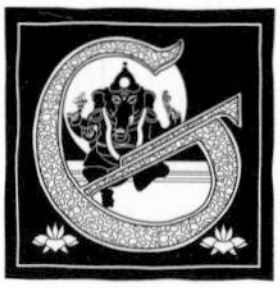

Gaṇeśa: गणेश "Lord of Categories." Or: "Lord of attendants *(gaṇa),*" synonymous with *Gaṇapati.* Gaṇeśa is a Mahādeva, the beloved elephant-faced Deity honored by Hindus of every sect.

Gaṇeśa Chaturthī: गणेश चतुर्थी The birthday of Lord Gaṇeśa, a ten-day festival of August-September that culminates in a parade called Gaṇeśa Visarjana. It is a time of rejoicing, when all Hindus worship together.

God: Supernal being. Either the Supreme God, Śiva, or one of the Mahādevas, great souls, who are among His creation.

Goddess: Female representation or manifestation of Divinity; Śakti or Devī. *Goddess* can refer to a female perception or depiction of a causal-plane being (Mahādeva) in its natural state, which is genderless, or it can refer to an astral-plane being residing in a female astral body.

Gods: Mahādevas, "great beings of light." In *Dancing with Śiva,* the plural form of *God* refers to extremely advanced beings existing in their self-effulgent soul bodies in the causal plane.

Gorakshanatha (Gorakshanātha): गोरक्षनाथ Profound *siddha yoga* master of the Ādinātha Sampradāya (ca 950). Expounder and foremost *guru* of Siddha Siddhānta Śaivism. He traveled and extolled the greatness of Śiva throughout North India and Nepal where he and his *guru,* Matsyendranatha, are still highly revered.

God Realization: Direct and personal experience of the Divine within oneself. It can refer to either 1) *savikalpa samādhi* ("enstasy with form") in its various levels, from the experience of inner light to the realization of Satchidānanda, pure consciousness, or 2) *nirvikalpa samādhi* ("enstasy without form"), union with the transcendent Absolute, Paraśiva, the Self God, beyond time, form and space. In *Yoga's Forgotten Foundation,* the expression *God Realization* is used to name both of the above *samādhis,* whereas *Self Realization* refers only to *nirvikalpa samādhi.*

grace: "Benevolence, love, giving," from the Latin *gratia,* "favor," "goodwill." God's power of revealment, *anugraha śakti* ("kindness, showing favor"), by which souls are awakened to their true, Divine nature. Grace in the unripe stages of the spiritual journey is experienced by the devotee as receiving gifts or boons, often unbidden, from God. The mature soul finds himself surrounded by grace. He sees all of God's actions as grace, whether they be seemingly pleasant and helpful or not. Grace is not only the force of illumination or revealment. It also includes Śiva's other four powers—creation, preservation, destruction and concealment—through which He provides the world of experience and limits the soul's consciousness so that it may evolve. More broadly, grace is God's ever-flowing love and compassion, *kāruṇya,* also known as *kṛipā* ("tenderness, compassion") and *prasāda* (literally, "clearness, purity"). The concealment power is known as veiling grace, God's power to obscure the soul's divine nature, or *tirodhāna śakti,* the particular energy of Śiva that binds the three bonds of *āṇava, karma, māyā* to the soul. It is a purposeful limiting of consciousness to give the opportunity to the soul to grow and mature through experience of the world.

guṇa: गुण "Strand; quality." The three constituent principles of *prakṛiti,* primal nature. The three *guṇas* are ***—sattva:*** Quiescent, rarified, translucent, pervasive, reflecting the light of Pure Consciousness. ***—rajas:*** "Passion," inherent in energy, movement, action, emotion, life. ***—tamas:*** "Darkness," inertia, density, the force of contraction, resistance and dissolution.

guru: गुरु "Weighty one," indicating an authority of great knowledge or skill. A teacher or guide in any subject, such as music, dance, sculpture, but especially religion. Often preceded by a qualifying prefix. Hence, *kulaguru* (family teacher), *vīnaguru (vīṇa* teacher) and *satguru* (spiritual preceptor). In astrology, *guru* names the planet Jupiter, also known as Bṛihaspati. According to the *Advayatāraka Upanishad* (14–18), *guru* means "dispeller *(gu)* of darkness *(ru).*"

guru paramparā: गुरुपरंपरा "Preceptorial succession" (literally, "from one to another"). A line of spiritual *gurus* in authentic succession of initiation; the chain of mystical power and authorized continuity, passed from *guru* to *guru.* Cf: *sampradāya.*

guru-śishya system: गुरुशिष्य "Master-disciple system." An important education system of Hinduism whereby the teacher conveys his knowledge and tradition to a student. Such knowledge, whether it be Vedic-Āgamic art, architecture or spirituality, is imparted through the developing relationship between *guru* and disciple.

haṭha yoga: हठयोग "Forceful yoga." A system of physical and mental exercise developed in ancient times as a means of rejuvenation by *ṛishis* and *tapasvins,* used today in preparing the body and mind for meditation.

Haṭha Yoga Pradīpikā: हठयोगप्रदीपिका "Elucidation of_*haṭha yoga.*" A 14th-century text of 389 verses by Svatmarama Yogin that describes the philosophy and practices of *haṭha yoga.*

heart *chakra:* *Anāhata chakra.* Center of direct cognition. See: *chakra.*

hiṁsā: हिंसा "Injury; harm; hurt." Injuriousness, hostility—mental, verbal or physical. See: *ahiṁsā.*

Hindu: हिन्दु A follower of, or relating to, Hinduism. See: *Hinduism.*

Hinduism (Hindu Dharma): हिन्दुधर्म India's indigenous religious and cultural system, followed today by nearly one billion adherents, mostly in India, but with the large diaspora in many other countries. Also called Sanātana Dharma, "Eternal Religion" and Vaidika Dharma, "Religion of the *Vedas.*" It is a family of myriad faiths with four primary denominations: Śaivism, Vaishṇavism, Śāktism and Smārtism.

homa: होम "Fire-offering." A ceremony of offering oblations to the Gods through the medium of fire in a sanctified fire pit, *homakuṇḍa,* usually made of earthen bricks. *Homa* rites are enjoined in the *Vedas, Āgamas* and *Dharma* and *Gṛihya Śāstras.*

hrī: ह्री "Remorse; modesty." See: *yama-niyama.*

iḍā nāḍī: इडानाडी "Soothing channel." The feminine psychic current flowing along the spine. See: *kuṇḍalinī, nāḍī.*

instinctive: "Natural" or "innate." From the Latin *instinctus,* "impelling, instigating." The drives and impulses that order the animal world and the physical and lower *astral* aspects of humans—for example, self-preservation, procreation, hunger and thirst, as well as the emotions of greed, hatred, anger, fear, lust and jealousy.

instinctive mind: *Manas chitta.* The lower mind, which controls the basic faculties of perception, movement, as well as ordinary thought and emotion.

internalized worship: *Yoga.* Worship or contact with God and Gods via meditation and contemplation rather than through external ritual.

intuition (to intuit): Direct understanding or cognition, which bypasses the process of reason.

invocation (to invoke): A "calling or summoning," as to a God, saint, etc., for blessings and assistance. Also, a formal prayer or chant. See: *mantra.*

Iraivan: இறைவன் "Worshipful one; divine one." One of the most ancient Tamil appellations for God. See: *San Marga Sanctuary.*

Iraivan Temple: See: *San Marga Sanctuary.*

irul: இருள் "Darkness." The first of three stages of the *sakala avasthai* where the soul's impetus is toward *pāśa-jñānam,* knowledge and experience of the world. See: *pāśa-jñānam, sakala avasthā.*

iruvinaioppu: இருவினையொப்பு "Balance." The balance which emerges in the life of a soul in the stage of *marul,* or *paśu-jñānam,* the second stage of the *sakala avasthai,* when the soul turns toward the good and holy, becomes centered within himself, unaffected by the ups and downs in life. See: *marul, paśu-jñānam, sakala avasthā.*

Īśvarapūjana: ईश्वरपूजन "Worship." See: *yama-niyama.*

jagadāchārya: जगदाचार्य "World teacher."

japa: जप "Recitation." Concentrated repeating of a *mantra,* silently or aloud, often counting on a *mālā* or strand of beads. A cure for pride and arrogance, jealousy, fear and confusion.

jīva: जीव "Living, existing." From *jīv,* "to live." The individual soul, *ātman,* during its embodied state, bound by the three *malas (āṇava, karma* and *māyā).*

jñāna: ज्ञान "Knowledge; wisdom." The matured state of the soul. It is the wisdom that comes as an aftermath of the *kuṇḍalinī* breaking through the door of *Brahman* into the realization of Paraśiva, Absolute Reality. *Jñāna* is the awakened, superconscious state *(kāraṇa chitta)* flowing into daily life situations.

jñāna dāna: ज्ञानदान "Gifts of wisdom." The *karma yoga* of printing, sponsoring and distributing Hindu religious literature, pamphlets and books, free of charge as a way of helping others spiritually.

jñānī: ज्ञानी "Sage." Possessing *jñāna.* See: *jñāna.*

jyotisha: ज्योतिष From *jyoti,* "light." "The science of the lights (or stars)," Hindu astrology, analyzing events and circumstances, delineating character and determining auspicious moments, according to the positions and movements of heavenly bodies.

Kailasa (Kailāsa): कैलास "Crystalline" or "abode of bliss." The Himalayan peak in Western Tibet; the earthly abode of Lord Śiva, a pilgrimage destination for Hindus and Tibetan Buddhists.

Kailāsa Paramparā: कैलासपरंपरा A spiritual lineage of 163 *siddhas*, a major stream of the Nandinātha Sampradāya, proponents of the ancient philosophy of monistic Śaiva Siddhānta. The first of these masters that history recalls was Maharishi Nandinatha (or Nandikesvara) 2,250 years ago, *satguru* to the great Tirumular, ca 200 BCE, and seven other disciples (as stated in the *Tirumantiram).* The lineage continued down the centuries and is alive today—the first recent *siddha* known being the "Rishi from the Himalayas," so named because he descended from those holy mountains. In South India, he initiated Kadaitswami (ca 1810–1875), who in turn initiated Chellappaswami (1840–1915). Chellappan passed the mantle of authority to Sage Yogaswami (1872–1964), who in 1949 initiated Sivaya Subramuniyaswami (1927–2001), who in 2001 ordained the current preceptor, Satguru Bodhinatha Veylanswami (1942–). See: *Nātha Sampradāya.*

Kali Yuga: कलियुग "Dark Age." The Kali Yuga is the last age in the repetitive cycle of four phases of time our solar system passes through. It is comparable to the darkest part of the night, as the forces of ignorance are in full power and many subtle faculties of the soul are obscured.

karma: कर्म "Action," "deed." 1) any act or deed; 2) the principle of cause and effect; 3) a consequence or "fruit of action" *(karmaphala)* or "after effect" *(uttaraphala),* which sooner or later returns upon the doer. What we sow, we shall reap in this or future lives. Selfish, hateful acts *(pāpakarma* or *kukarma)* will bring suffering. Benevolent actions *(puṇyakarma* or *sukarma)* will bring loving reactions. *Karma* is threefold: *sañchita, prārabdha* and *kriyamāna.* **—*sañchita karma:*** "Accumulated actions." The sum of all *karmas* of this life and past lives. **—*prārabdha karma:*** "Actions begun; set in motion." That portion of *sañchita karma* that is bearing fruit and shaping the events and conditions of the current life, including the nature of one's bodies, personal tendencies and associations. **—*kriyamāna karma:*** "Being made."

karma yoga: कर्मयोग "Union through action." Selfless service.

Kauai Aadheenam: Monastery-temple complex founded by Sivaya Subramuniyaswami in 1970; international headquarters of Saiva Siddhanta Church.

kośa: कोश "Sheath; vessel, container; layer." Philosophically, five sheaths through which the soul functions simultaneously in the various planes or levels of existence. The *kośas* are **—*annamaya kośa:*** "Sheath composed of food." The physical or odic body, coarsest of sheaths in comparison to the faculties of the soul, yet indispensable for evolution and Self Realization, because only within it can all fourteen *chakras* fully function. See: *chakra.* **—*prāṇamaya kośa:*** "Sheath composed of *prāṇa* (vital force)." The *prāṇic* or health body, or the etheric body or etheric double, coexisting within the physical body as its source of life, breath and vitality, and is its connection with the astral body. *Prāṇa* moves in the *prāṇamaya kośa* as five primary currents or *vayus,* "vital airs or winds." *Prāṇamaya kośa* disintegrates at death along with the physical body. See: *prāṇa* **—*manomaya kośa:*** "Mind-formed sheath." The lower astral body, from *manas,* "thought, will, wish." The instinctive-intellectual sheath of ordinary thought, desire and emotion. The *manomaya kośa* takes form as the physical body develops and is discarded in the inner worlds before rebirth. **—*vijñānamaya kośa:*** "Sheath of cognition." The mental or cognitive-intuitive sheath, also called the actinodic sheath. It is the vehicle of higher thought, *vijñāna*—understanding, knowing, direct cognition, wisdom, intuition and creativity. ***—ānandamaya kośa:*** "Body of bliss." The intuitive-superconscious sheath or actinic-causal body. The inmost soul form *(svarūpa),* the ultimate foundation of all life, intelligence and higher faculties. Its essence is Parāśakti (Pure Consciousness) and Paraśiva (the Absolute). It is the soul itself, a body of light, also called *kāraṇa śarīra,* causal body, and *karmāśaya,* holder of *karmas* of this and all past lives. *Kāraṇa chitta,* "causal mind," names the soul's superconscious mind, of which Parāśakti (or Satchidānanda) is the rarified substratum.

kevala avasthā: केवल अवस्था "Stage of oneness, aloneness." (Tamil: *avasthai.)* In Śaiva Siddhānta, the first of three stages of the soul's evolution, a state beginning with its emanation or spawning by Lord Śiva as an etheric form unaware of itself, a spark of the Divine shrouded in a cloud of darkness known as *āṇava.* Here the soul is likened to a seed hidden in the ground, yet to germinate and unfold its potential. See: *sakala avasthā, śuddha avasthā.*

kriyā: क्रिया "Action." 1) Doing of any kind. Specifically, religious action, especially rites or ceremonies. 2) Involuntary physical movements occuring during meditation that are pretended or caused by lack of emotional self-control or by the premature or unharnessed arousal of the *kuṇḍalinī.* 3) *Haṭha yoga* techniques for cleansing the mucous membranes. 4) The second stage of the Śaiva path, religious action, *kriyā pāda.* See: *pāda.*

kriyā mārga: क्रियामार्ग See *kriyā pāda.*

kriyā pāda: क्रियापाद् "Stage of religious action; worship." The stage of worship and devotion, second of four progressive stages of maturation on the Śaiva Siddhānta path of attainment. See: *pāda.*

kshamā: क्षमा "Forebearance." See: *yama-niyama.*

kuṇḍalinī: कुण्डलिनी "She who is coiled; serpent power." The primordial cosmic energy in every individual which, at first, lies coiled like a serpent at the base of the spine and eventually, through the practice of *yoga,* rises up the *sushumṇā nāḍī.* As it rises, the *kuṇḍalinī* awakens each successive *chakra. Nirvikalpa samādhi,* enlightenment, comes as it pierces through the door of Brahman at the core of the *sahasrāra* and enters! *Kuṇḍalinī śakti* then returns to rest in any one of the seven *chakras.* Śivasāyujya is complete when the *kuṇḍalinī* arrives back in the *sahasrāra* and remains coiled in this crown *chakra.*

kuṇḍalinī yoga: कुण्डलिनीयोग "Uniting the serpent power." Advanced meditative practices and *sādhana* techniques, a part of *rāja yoga,* performed to deliberately arouse the *kuṇḍalinī* power and guide it up the spine into the crown *chakra, sahasrāra.* In its highest form, this *yoga* is the natural result of *sādhanas* and *tapas* well performed, rather than a distinct system of striving and teaching in its own right.

liberal Hinduism: A synonym for Smārtism and the closely related neo-Indian religion. See: *neo-Indian religion, Smārtism.*

liberation: *Moksha,* release from the bonds of *pāśa,* after which the soul is liberated from *saṁsāra* (the round of births and deaths). In Śaiva Siddhānta, *pāśa* is the threefold bondage of *āṇava, karma* and *māyā,* which limit and confine the soul to the reincarnational cycle so that it may evolve. *Moksha* is freedom from the fettering power of these bonds, which do not cease to exist, but no longer have the power to fetter or bind the soul.

loka: लोक "World, habitat, realm, or plane of existence." From *loc,* "to shine, be bright, visible." A dimension of manifest existence; cosmic region. Each *loka* reflects or involves a particular range of consciousness. The three primary *lokas* are 1) **—Bhūloka:** "Earth world." The world perceived through the five senses, also called the gross plane, as it is the most dense of the worlds. 2) **—Antarloka:** "Inner or in-between world." Known in English as the subtle or astral plane, the intermediate dimension between the physical and causal worlds, where souls in their astral bodies sojourn between incarnations and when they sleep. 3) **—Śivaloka:** "World of Śiva," and of the Gods and highly evolved souls. The causal plane, also called Kāraṇaloka, existing deep within the Antarloka at a higher level of vibration, it is a world of superconsciousness and extremely refined energy. It is the plane of creativity and intuition, the quantum level of the universe, where souls exists in self-effulgent bodies made of actinic particles of light. It is here that God and Gods move and lovingly guide the evolution of all the worlds and shed their ever-flowing grace. See: *three worlds.*

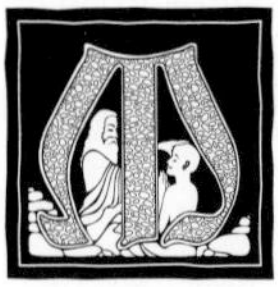

Mahādeva: महादेव "Great shining one; God." Referring either to God Śiva or any of the highly evolved beings who live in the Śivaloka in their natural, effulgent soul bodies.

mahāsamādhi: महासमाधि "Great enstasy." The death, or giving up of the physical body, of a great soul, an event occasioned by tremendous blessings. Also names the shrine in which the remains of a great soul are entombed. See: *cremation, death.*

Mahāśivarātri: महाशिवरात्रि "Śiva's great night." Śaivism's foremost festival, celebrated on the night before the new moon in February-March. Fasting and an all-night vigil are observed as well as other disciplines: chanting, praying, meditating and worshiping Śiva as the Source and Self of all that exists.

mahātala chakra: महातल चक्र Sixth netherworld. Region of consciencelessness. See: *chakra.*

mala: मल "Impurity." An important term in Śaivism referring to three bonds, called *pāśa—āṇava, karma,* and *māyā*—which limit the soul, preventing it from knowing its true, divine nature.

mālā: माला "Garland." A strand of beads for holy recitation, *japa,* usually made of *rudrāksha, tulasī,* sandalwood or crystal. Also a flower garland.

malaparipakam: மலபரிபாகம் "Ripening of bonds." The state attained after the three *malas, āṇava, karma* and *māyā,* are brought under control during *marul,* the second stage of the *sakala avasthai.* At this time, the Lord's concealing grace, *tirodhāna śakti,* has accomplished its work, giving way to *anugraha,* His revealing grace, leading to the descent of grace, *śaktinipāta.* See: *sakala avasthā, śaktinipāta.*

maṇipūra chakra: मणिपूरचक्र "Wheeled city of jewels." Solar-plexus center of willpower. See: *chakra.*

mānsāhāra: मांसाहार "Meat-eating."

mānsāhārī: मांसाहारी "Meat-eater." One who follows a nonvegetarian diet. See: *vegetarian.*

mantra: मन्त्र "Mystic formula." A sound, syllable, word or phrase endowed with special power, usually drawn from scripture.

marul: மருள் "Confusion." The second of the three stages of the *sakala avasthai* when the soul is "caught" between the world and God and begins to seek knowledge of its own true nature, *paśu-jñānam*. See: *paśu-jñānam, sakala avasthā.*

***mati:* मति** "Cognition, understanding; conviction." See: *yama-niyama.*

***mauna:* मौन** The discipline of remaining silent.

***māyā:* माया** "She who measures;" or "mirific energy." The substance emanated from Śiva through which the world of form is manifested. Hence all creation is also termed *māyā*. It is the cosmic creative force, the principle of manifestation, ever in the process of creation, preservation and dissolution.

meditation: *Dhyāna*. Sustained concentration. Meditation describes a quiet, alert, powerfully concentrated state wherein new knowledge and insights are awakened from within as awareness focuses one-pointedly on an object or specific line of thought.

mendicant: A beggar; a wandering monk who lives on alms.

mental body (sheath): The higher-mind layer of the subtle or astral body in which the soul functions in the Maharloka of the Antarloka or subtle plane. In Sanskrit, the mental body is *vijñānamaya kośa*, "sheath of cognition." See: *kośa, subtle body.*

mental plane: Names the refined strata of the subtle world. In Sanskrit, it is called Maharloka or Devaloka, realm of *anāhata chakra*. Here the soul is shrouded in the mental or cognitive sheath, *vijñānamaya kośa.*

metaphysics: 1) The branch of philosophy dealing with first causes and nature of reality. 2) The science of mysticism.

mind (three phases): A perspective of mind as instinctive, intellectual and superconscious. **—instinctive mind.** *Manas chitta*, the seat of desire and governor of sensory and motor organs. **—intellectual mind.** *Buddhi chitta*, the faculty of thought and intelligence. **—superconscious mind:** *Kāraṇa chitta*, the strata of intuition, benevolence and spiritual sustenance. Its most refined essence is Parāsakti, or Satchidānanda, all-knowing, omnipresent consciousness, the One transcendental, self-luminous, divine mind common to all souls.

mind (five states): A view of the mind in five parts. **—conscious mind:** *Jāgrat chitta* ("wakeful consciousness"). The ordinary, waking, thinking state of mind. **—subconscious mind:** *Saṁskāra chitta* ("impression mind"). The part of mind "beneath" the conscious mind, the storehouse or recorder of all experience (whether remembered consciously or not)—the holder of past impressions, reactions and desires. Also, the seat of involuntary physiological processes. **—subsubconscious mind:** *Vāsanā chitta* ("mind of subliminal traits"). The area of the subconscious mind formed when two thoughts or experiences of the same rate of intensity are sent into the subconscious at different times and, intermingling, give rise to a new and totally different rate of vibration. **—superconscious mind:** *Kāraṇa chitta*. The mind of light, the all-knowing intelligence of the soul. At its deepest level, the superconscious is Parāśakti, or Satchidānanda, the Divine Mind of God Śiva. **—subsuperconscious mind:** *Anukāraṇa chitta*. The superconscious mind working through the conscious and subconscious states, which brings forth intuition, clarity and insight.

***mitāhāra:* मिताहार** "Measured eating; moderate appetite," a requisite for good health and success in *yoga*. An ideal portion per meal is one a *kuḍava*,no more than would fill the two hands held side by side and slightly cupped piled high. See: *yama-niyama.*

***moksha:* मोक्ष** "Liberation." Release from transmigration, *saṁsāra*, the round of births and deaths, which occurs after *karma* has been resolved and *nirvikalpa samādhi*—realization of the Self, Paraśiva—has been attained. Same as *mukti.*

monism: "Doctrine of oneness." 1) The philosophical view that there is only one ultimate substance or principle. 2) The view that reality is a unified whole without independent parts. See: *dvaita-advaita.*

monistic theism: Advaita Īśvaravāda. The doctrine that reality is a one whole or existence without independent parts, coupled with theism, the belief that God exists as a real, conscious, personal Supreme Being—two perspectives ordinarily considered contradictory or mutually exclusive, since theism implies dualism.

mukti: मुक्ति "Release," "liberation." A synonym for *moksha.*

mūlādhāra chakra: मूलाधारचक्र "Root-support wheel." Four-petaled psychic center at the base of the spine; governs memory. See: *chakra.*

mūrti: मूर्ति "Form; manifestation, embodiment, personification." An image, icon or effigy of God or a God used during worship.

Murugan: முருகன் "Beautiful one," a favorite name of Kārttikeya among the Tamils of South India, Sri Lanka and elsewhere.

nāḍī: नाडी "Conduit; river." A nerve fiber or energy channel of the subtle (inner) bodies of man. It is said there are 72,000 *nāḍīs.* These interconnect the *chakras.* The three main *nāḍīs* are *iḍā, piṅgalā* and *sushumṇā.* ***—iḍā,*** also known as *chandra* (moon) *nāḍī,* is pink in color. Its flows downward, ending on the left side of the body. This current is feminine in nature and is the channel of physical-emotional energy. ***—piṅgalā,*** also known as *sūrya* (sun) *nāḍī,* is blue in color. It flows upward, ending on the right side of the body. This current is masculine in nature and is the channel of intellectual-mental energy. ***—sushumṇā*** is the major nerve current which passes through the spinal column from the *mūlādhāra chakra* at the base to the *sahasrāra* at the crown of the head. It is the channel of *kuṇḍalinī.*

Namaḥ Śivāya: नमः शिवाय "Adoration (homage) to Śiva." The supreme *mantra* of Śaivism, known as the *Pañchākshara,* or "five syllables."

namaskāra: नमस्कार "Reverent salutations." Traditional Hindu verbal greeting and *mudrā* where the palms are joined together and held before the heart or raised to the level of the forehead. The *mudrā* is also called *añjali.* It is a devotional gesture made equally before a temple Deity, holy person, friend or even momentary acquaintance.

Nandinātha Sampradāya: नन्दिनाथसंप्रदाय See: *Nātha Sampradāya.*

Narakaloka: नरकलोक Abode of darkness. Literally, "pertaining to man." The nether worlds. Equivalent to the Western term *hell,* a gross region of the Antarloka. Naraka is a congested, distressful area where demonic beings and young souls may sojourn until they resolve the darksome *karmas* they have created. Here beings suffer the consequences of their own misdeeds in previous lives. Naraka is understood as having seven regions, called *tala,* corresponding to the states of consciousness of the seven lower *chakras.*

Natchintanai: நற்சிந்தனை The collected songs of Sage Yogaswami (1872-1964) of Jaffna, Sri Lanka, extolling the power of the *satguru,* worship of Lord Śiva, adherance to the path of *dharma* and striving for the attainment of Self Realization. See: *Kailāsa Paramparā, Yogaswami.*

Nātha: नाथ "Master, lord; adept." An ancient Himalayan tradition of Śaiva-yoga mysticism whose first historically known exponent was Nandikeśvara (ca 250 BCE). *Nātha*—Self-Realized adept—designates the extraordinary ascetic masters (or devotees) of this school.

Nātha Sampradāya: नाथसंप्रदाय "Traditional doctrine of knowledge of masters," a philosophical and *yogic* tradition of Śaivism whose origins are unknown. This oldest of Śaivite *sampradāyas* existing today consists of two major streams: the Nandinātha and the Ādinātha. The Nandinātha Sampradāya has had as exemplars Maharishi Nandinatha and his disciples: Patanjali (author of the *Yoga Sūtras)* and Tirumular (author of *Tirumantiram).* Among its representatives today are the successive *siddhars* of the Kailāsa Paramparā. The Ādinātha lineage's known exemplars are Maharishi Adinatha, Matsyendranatha and Gorakshanatha, who founded a well-known order of *yogīs.* See: *Kailāsa Paramparā.*

neo: A prefix meaning new and different; modified.

neo-Indian religion: *Navabhārata Dharma.* A modern form of liberal Hinduism that carries forward basic Hindu cultural values—such as dress, diet and the arts—while allowing religious values to subside. It emerged after the British Rāj, when India declared itself an independent, secular state. It was cultivated by the Macaulay education system, implanted in India by the British, which aggressively undermined Hindu thought and belief. Neo-Indian religion encourages Hindus to follow any combination of theological, scriptural, *sādhana* and worship patterns, regardless of sectarian or religious origin. Extending out of and beyond the Smārta system of worshiping the Gods of each major sect, it incorporates holy icons from all religions, including Jesus, Mother Mary and Buddha. Many *Navabhāratis* choose to not call themselves Hindus but to declare themselves members of all the world's religions. See: *Smārtism.*

New Age: According to *Webster's New World Dictionary:* "Of or pertaining to a cultural movement popular in the 1980s [and 90s] characterized by a concern with spiritual consciousness, and variously combining belief in reincarnation and astrology with such practices as meditation, vegetarianism and holistic medicine."

nirvikalpa samādhi: निर्विकल्पसमाधि "Undifferentiated trance, enstasy *(samādhi)* without form or seed." The realization of the Self, Paraśiva, a state of oneness beyond all change or diversity; beyond time, form and space. See: *samādhi.*

niyama: नियम "Restraint." See: *yama-niyama.*

pada: पद् "A step, pace, stride; footstep, trace."

pāda: पाद् "The foot (of men and animals); quarter-part, section; stage; path." Names the major sections of the Āgamic texts and the corresponding stages of practice and unfoldment on the path to *moksha.* According to Śaiva Siddhānta, there are four *pādas,* which are successive and cumulative; i.e. in accomplishing each one the soul prepares itself for the next. —***charyā pāda:*** "Good conduct stage." Learning to live righteously, serve selflessly, performing *karma yoga.* —***kriyā pāda:*** "Religious action; worship stage." Stage of *bhakti yoga,* of cultivating devotion through performing *pūjā* and regular daily *sādhana.* —***yoga pāda:*** Having matured in the *charyā* and *kriyā pādas,* the soul now turns to internalized worship and *rāja yoga* under the guidance of a *satguru.* —***jñāna pāda:*** "Stage of wisdom." Once the soul has attained Realization, it is henceforth a wise one who lives out the life of the body, shedding blessings on mankind.

paṇḍara: पण्डर An informal order of independent priests, often self-taught and self-appointed, who emerge within a community to perform *pūjās* at a sacred tree, a simple shrine or a temple.

pandit (paṇḍita): पण्डित (Also, *pundit.)* A Hindu religious scholar or theologian, well versed in philosophy, liturgy, religious law and sacred science.

pāpa: पाप "Wickedness; sin, crime." 1) Bad or evil. 2) Wrongful action. 3) Demerit earned through wrongdoing. Each act of *pāpa* carries its *karmic* consequence, *karmaphala,* "fruit of action," for which scriptures delineate specific penance for expiation. *Pāpa* can produce disease, depression, loneliness and such, but can be dissolved through penance *(prāyaśchitta),* austerity *(tapas)* and good deeds *(sukṛityā).*

paramparā: परंपरा "Uninterrupted succession." A lineage.

parārtha pūjā: परार्थपूजा "Public liturgy and worship." See: *pūjā.*

Paraśiva: परशिव "Transcendent Śiva." The Self God, Śiva's first perfection, Absolute Reality. Paraśiva is *That* which is beyond the grasp of consciousness, transcends time, form and space and defies description. To merge with the Absolute in mystic union is the ultimate goal of all incarnated souls, the reason for their living on this planet, and the deepest meaning of their experiences. Attainment of this is called Self Realization or *nirvikalpa samādhi.*

pāśa: पाश "Tether; noose." The whole of existence, manifest and unmanifest. That which binds or limits the soul and keeps it (for a time) from manifesting its full potential. *Pāśa* consists of the soul's threefold bondage of *āṇava, karma* and *māyā.* See: *Pati-paśu-pāśa.*

paśu: पशु "Cow, cattle, kine; fettered individual." Refers to animals or beasts, including man. In philosophy, the soul. Śiva as lord of creatures is called Paśupati. See: *Pati-paśu-pāśa.*

pātāla chakra: पाताल चक्र "Fallen" or "sinful region." The seventh *chakra* below the *mūlādhāra,* centered in the soles of the feet. Corresponds to the seventh and lowest astral netherworld beneath the earth's surface, called Kākola ("black poison") or Pātāla. This is the realm in which misguided souls indulge in destruction for the sake of destruction, of torture, and of murder for the sake of murder. *Pātāla* also names the netherworld in general, and is a synonym for *Naraka.* See: *chakra, loka, Narakaloka.*

Patanjali (Patañjali): पतञ्जलि A Śaivite Nātha *siddha* (ca 200 BCE) who codified the ancient *yoga* philosophy which outlines the path to enlightenment through purification, control and transcendence of the mind.

Pati: पति "Master; lord; owner." A name for God Śiva indicating His commanding relationship with souls as caring ruler and helpful guide. See: *Pati-paśu-pāśa.*

Pati-jñānam: பதிஞானம் "Knowledge of God," sought for by the soul in the third stage of the *sakala avasthai,* called *arul.* See: *arul, sakala avasthā, śaktinipāta.*

Pati-paśu-pāśa: पति पशु पाश Literally: "master, cow and tether." These are the three primary elements of Śaiva Siddhānta philosophy: God, soul and world—Divinity, man and cosmos—seen as a mystically and intricately interrelated unity. Pati is God, envisioned as a cowherd. *Paśu* is the soul, envisioned as a cow. *Pāśa* is the all-important force or fetter by which God brings souls along the path to Truth.

paśu-jñānam: பசுஞானம் "Soul-knowledge." The object of seeking in the second stage of the *sakala avasthai,* called *marul.* See: *marul, sakala avasthā.*

payasam: பாயாசம் A cooked, milk-based pudding dessert often served at special festive occasions, generally made from tapioca or rice.

penance: *Prāyaśchitta.* Atonement, expiation. An act of devotion *(bhakti),* austerity *(tapas)* or discipline *(sukṛitya)* undertaken to soften or nullify the anticipated reaction to a past action.

pilgrimage: *Tīrthayātrā.* Journeying to a holy temple, near or far, performed by all Hindus at least once each year. See: *tīrthayātrā.*

piṅgalā: **पिंगला** "Tawny channel." The masculine psychic current flowing along the spine. See: *nāḍī.*

prāṇa: **प्राण** Vital energy or life principle. Literally, "vital air," from the root *praṇ,* "to breathe." *Prāṇa* in the human body moves in the *prāṇamaya kośa* as five primary life currents known as *vāyus,* "vital airs or winds." *Prāṇa* sometimes denotes the power or animating force of the cosmos, the sum total of all energy and forces.

Praṇava: **प्रणव** "Humming." The *mantra Aum,* denoting God as the Primal Sound. It can be heard as the sound of one's own nerve system, like the sound of an electrical transformer or a swarm of bees. The meditator is taught to inwardly transform this sound into the inner light which lights the thoughts, and bask in this blissful consciousness. *Praṇava* is also known as the sound of the *nādanāḍī śakti.* See: *Aum.*

prāṇāyāma: **प्राणायाम** "Breath control." Science of controlling *prāṇa* through breathing techniques in which the lengths of inhalation, retention and exhalation are modulated. *Prāṇāyāma* prepares the mind for meditation. See: *ashṭaṅga yoga.*

prāṇic body: The subtle, life-giving sheath called *prāṇamaya kośa.* See: *kośa.*

prārabdha karma: **प्रारब्धकर्म** "Action that has been unleashed or aroused." See: *karma.*

prasāda: **प्रसाद** "Clarity, brightness; grace." 1) The virtue of serenity and graciousness. 2) Food offered to the Deity or the *guru,* or the blessed remnants of such food. 3) Any propitiatory offering.

pratyāhāra: **प्रत्याहार** "Withdrawal." The drawing in of forces. In *yoga,* the withdrawal from external consciousness. (Also a synonym for *pralaya.)* See: *ashṭaṅga yoga.*

prāyaśchitta: **प्रायश्चित्त** "Predominant thought or aim." Penance. Acts of atonement. See: *penance.*

protocol: Customs of proper etiquette and ceremony, especially in relation to religious or political dignitaries.

pūjā: **पूजा** "Worship, adoration." An Āgamic rite of worship performed in the home, temple or shrine, to the *mūrti, śrī pādukā,* or other consecrated object, or to a person, such as the *satguru.* Its inner purpose is to purify the atmosphere around the object worshiped, establish a connection with the inner worlds and invoke the presence of God, Gods or one's *guru. Ātmārtha pūjā* is done for oneself and immediate family, usually at home in a private shrine. *Parārtha pūjā* is public *pūjā,* performed by authorized or ordained priests in a public shrine or temple.

pujārī: **पुजारी** "Worshiper." A general term for Hindu temple priests, as well as anyone performing *pūjā.*

puṇya: **पुण्य** "Holy; virtuous; auspicious." 1) Good or righteous. 2) Meritorious action. 3) Merit earned through right thought, word and action. *Puṇya* includes all forms of doing good, from the simplest helpful deed to a lifetime of conscientious beneficence. *Puṇya* produces inner contentment, deep joy, the feeling of security and fearlessness. See: *pāpa.*

purusha: **पुरुष** "The spirit that dwells in the body/in the universe." Person; spirit; man. Metaphysically, the soul, neither male nor female. Also used in Yoga and Sāṅkhya for the transcendent Self. A synonym for *ātman. Purusha* can also refer to the Supreme Being or Soul, as it sometimes does in the *Upanishads.* In Śaiva cosmology, *purusha* is the 25th of 36 *tattvas,* one level subtler than *prakṛiti.*

purusha dharma: **पुरुषधर्म** "A man's code of duty and conduct." See: *dharma.*

R

rajas: रजस् "Passion; activity." See: *guṇa.*

rasātala chakra: रसातल चक्र "Subterranean region." The fifth *chakra* below the *mūlādhāra,* centered in the ankles. Corresponds to the fifth astral netherworld beneath the earth's surface, called Ṛijīsha ("expelled") or Rasātala. Region of selfishness, self-centeredness and possessiveness. *Rasā* means "earth, soil; moisture." See: *chakra, Narakaloka.*

reincarnation: "Re-entering the flesh." *Punarjanma;* metempsychosis. The process wherein souls take on a physical body through the birth process.

renunciation: See: *sannyāsa.*

restraints: See: *yama-niyama.*

revealing grace: See: *anugraha śakti, grace.*

ṛishi: ऋषि "Seer." A term for an enlightened being, emphasizing psychic perception and visionary wisdom.

rudrāksha: रुद्राक्ष "Eye of Rudra; or red-eyed." Refers to the third eye, or *ājñā chakra.* Marble-sized, multi-faced, reddish-brown seeds from the *Eleocarpus ganitrus,* or blue marble tree, which are sacred to Śiva and a symbol of His compassion for humanity.

S

sacrament: 1) Holy rite, especially one solemnized in a formal, consecrated manner which is a bonding between the recipient and God, Gods or *guru.* This includes rites of passage *(saṁskāra),* ceremonies sanctifying crucial events or stages of life. 2) *Prasāda.* Sacred substances, grace-filled gifts, blessed in sacred ceremony or by a holy person. See: *saṁskāra.*

sādhaka: साधक "Accomplished one; a devotee who performs *sādhana.*" A serious aspirant who has undertaken spiritual disciplines, is usually celibate and under the guidance of a *guru.* He wears white and may be under vows, but is not a *sannyāsin.*

sādhana: साधन "Effective means of attainment." Religious or spiritual disciplines, such as *pūjā, yoga,* meditation, *japa,* fasting and austerity.

sādhu: साधु "Virtuous one; straight, unerring." A holy man dedicated to the search for God. A *sādhu* may or may not be a *yogī* or a *sannyāsin,* or be connected in any way with a *guru* or legitimate lineage. *Sādhus* usually have no fixed abode and travel unattached from place to place, often living on alms.

sahasrāra chakra: सहस्रारचक्र "Thousand-spoked wheel." The cranial psychic force center. See: *chakra.*

Śaiva: शैव Of or relating to Śaivism or its adherents, of whom there are about 400 million in the world today. Same as *Śaivite.* See: *Śaivism.*

Śaiva Āgamas: शैव आगम The sectarian revealed scriptures of the Śaivas. Strongly theistic, they identify Śiva as the Supreme Lord, immanent and transcendent. They are in two main divisions: the 64 *Kashmīr Śaiva Āgamas* and the 28 *Śaiva Siddhānta Āgamas.* The latter group are the fundamental sectarian scriptures of Śaiva Siddhānta.

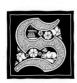

Śaiva Siddhānta: शैवसिद्धान्त "Final conclusions of Śaivism." The most widespread and influential Śaivite school today, predominant especially among the Tamil people of Sri Lanka and South India. It is the formalized theology of the divine revelations contained in the twenty-eight *Śaiva Āgamas.* For Śaiva Siddhāntins, Śiva is the totality of all, understood in three perfections: Parameśvara (the Personal Creator Lord), Parāśakti (the substratum of form) and Paraśiva (Absolute Reality which transcends all). Souls and world are identical in essence with Śiva, yet also differ in that they are evolving. A pluralistic stream arose in the middle ages from the teachings of Aghorasiva and Meykandar. See: *Śaivism.*

Śaivism (Śaiva): शैव The religion followed by those who worship Śiva as supreme God. Oldest of the four sects of Hinduism. The earliest historical evidence of Śaivism is from the 8,000-year-old Indus Valley civilization in the form of the famous seal of Śiva as Lord Paśupati, seated in a *yogic* pose. There are many schools of Śaivism, six of which are Śaiva Śiddhānta, Pāśupata Śaivism, Kashmīr Śaivism, Vīra Śaivism, Siddha Siddhānta and Śiva Advaita. They are based firmly on the *Vedas* and *Śaiva Āgamas,* and thus have much in common, including the following principle doctrines: 1) the five powers of Śiva—creation, preservation, destruction, revealing and concealing grace; 2) The three categories: Pati, *paśu* and *pāśa* ("God, souls and bonds"); 3) the three bonds: *āṇava, karma* and *māyā;* 4) the threefold power of Śiva: *icçhā śakti, kriyā śakti* and *jñāna śakti;* 5) the thirty-six *tattvas,* or categories of existence; 6) the need for initiation from a *satguru;* 7) the power of *mantra;* 8) the four *pādas* (stages): *charyā* (selfless service), *kriyā* (devotion), *yoga* (meditation), and *jñāna* (illumination)*;* 9) the belief in the Pañchākshara as the foremost *mantra,* and in *rudrāksha* and *vibhūti* as sacred aids to faith; 10) the beliefs in *satguru* (preceptor), Śivaliṅga (object of worship) and *saṅgama* (company of holy persons).

Śaivite (Śaiva): शैव Of or relating to Śaivism or its adherents, of whom there are about 400 million in the world today. See: *Śaivism.*

śākāhāra: शाकाहार "Vegetarian diet." From *śāka,* "vegetable;" and *āhāra,* "eating; taking food." See: *yama-niyama.*

sakala avasthā: सकल अवस्था "Stage of embodied being." (Tamil: *avasthai.)* In Śaiva Siddhānta, the second of three stages of the soul's evolution, when it is engaged in the world through the senses as it first develops a mental, then emotional and astral body, and finally a physical body, entering the cycles of birth, death and rebirth under the veiling powers of *karma* and *māya.* Progress through *sakala avasthā* is measured in three stages: 1) *irul,* "darkness;" when the impetus is toward *pāśa,* knowledge and experience of the world *(pāśa-jñānam)*; 2) *marul,* "confusion;" caught between the world and God, the soul begins to turn within for knowledge of its own nature *(paśu-jñānam)*; and 3) *arul,* "grace," when the soul seeks to know God (Pati-*jñānam*); and receive His grace. See: *avasthā.*

Śākta: शाक्त Of or relating to *Śāktism.* See: *Śāktism.*

Śakti: शक्ति "Power, energy." The active power or manifest energy of Śiva that pervades all of existence. Its most refined aspect is Parāśakti, or Satchidānanda, the pure consciousness and primal substratum of all form. This pristine, divine energy unfolds as *icçhā śakti* (the power of desire, will, love), *kriyā śakti* (the power of action) and *jñāna śakti* (the power of wisdom, knowing), represented as the three prongs of Śiva's *triśūla,* or trident. From these arise the five powers of revealment, concealment, dissolution, preservation and creation. In Śaiva Siddhānta, Śiva is All, and His divine energy, Śakti, is inseparable from Him. This unity is symbolized in the image of Ardhanārīśvara, "half-female God." In popular, village Hinduism, the unity of Śiva and Śakti is replaced with the concept of Śiva and Śakti as separate entities. Śakti is represented as female, and Śiva as male. In Hindu temples, art and mythology, they are everywhere seen as the divine couple. Within the Śākta religion, the worship of the Goddess is paramount, in Her many fierce and benign forms. Śakti is most easily experienced by devotees as the sublime, bliss-inspiring energy that emanates from a holy person or sanctified Hindu temple. See: *Śāktism.*

śaktinipāta: शक्तिनिपात "Descent of grace," occuring during the advanced stage of the soul's evolution called *arul,* at the end of the *sakala avasthai. Śaktinipāta* is two-fold: the internal descent is recognized as a tremendous yearning for Śiva; the outer descent of grace is the appearance of a *satguru.* At this stage, the devotee increasingly wants to devote himself to all that is spiritual and holy. Same as *śaktipāta.* See: *sakala avasthā.*

Śāktism (Śākta): शाक्त "Doctrine of power." The religion followed by those who worship the Supreme as the Divine Mother—Śakti or Devī—in Her many forms, both gentle and fierce. Śāktism is one of the four primary sects of Hinduism. Śāktism's first historical signs are thousands of female statuettes dated ca 5500 BCE recovered at the Mehrgarh village in India. In philosophy and practice, Śāktism greatly resembles Śaivism, both faiths promulgating, for example, the same ultimate goals of *advaitic* union with Śiva and *moksha.* But Śāktas worship Śakti as the Supreme Being exclusively, as the dynamic aspect of Divinity, while Śiva is considered solely transcendent and is not worshiped. See: *Śakti.*

samādhi: समाधि "Enstasy," "standing within one's Self." "Sameness; contemplation; union, wholeness; completion, accomplishment." *Samādhi* is the state of true *yoga,* in which the meditator and the object of meditation are one. *Samādhi* is of two levels. The first is *savikalpa samādhi* ("enstasy with form" or "seed"), identification or oneness with the essence of an object. Its highest form is the realization of the primal substratum or pure consciousness, Satchidānanda. The second is *nirvikalpa samādhi* ("enstasy without form" or "seed"), identification with the Self, in which all modes of consciousness are transcended and Absolute Reality, Paraśiva, beyond time, form and space, is experienced.

samayam: சமயம் "Religion."

sampradāya: संप्रदाय "Tradition," "transmission;" a philosophical or religious doctrine or lineage. A living stream of tradition or theology within Hinduism, passed on by oral training and initiation. Each *sampradāya* is often represented by many *paramparās.*

saṁsāra: संसार "Flow." The phenomenal world. The cycle of birth, death and rebirth; the total pattern of successive earthly lives experienced by a soul.

saṁskāra: संस्कार "Impression, activator; sanctification, preparation." 1) The imprints left on the subconscious mind by experience (from this or previous lives), which then color all of life, one's nature, responses, states of mind, etc. 2) A sacrament or rite done to mark a significant transition of life.

Sanātana Dharma: सनातनधर्म "Eternal religion" or "Everlasting path." It is a traditional designation for the Hindu religion. See: *Hinduism.*

San Mārga: सन्मार्ग "True path." The straight, spiritual path leading to the ultimate goal, Self Realization, without detouring into unnecessary psychic exploration or pointless development of *siddhis. San Mārga* also names the *jñāna pāda.*

San Marga Sanctuary: A meditation *tīrtha* at the foot of the extinct volcano, Mount Waialeale, on Hawaii's Garden Island, Kauai. Founded in 1970, it is among the many public services of Saiva Siddhanta Church, one of America's senior Hindu religious institutions.

sannidhāna: सन्निधान "Nearness; proximity; provost; taking charge of." A title of heads of monasteries: Guru Mahāsannidhāna. See: *sānnidhya.*

sānnidhya: सान्निध्य "(Divine) presence; nearness, indwelling." The radiance and blessed presence of *śakti* within and around a temple or a holy person.

sannyāsa: संन्यास "Renunciation." "Throwing down or abandoning." *Sannyāsa* is the repudiation of the *dharma,* including the obligations and duties, of the householder and the acceptance of the even more demanding *dharma* of the renunciate.

sannyāsin: संन्यासिन् "Renouncer." One who has taken *sannyāsa dīkshā.* A Hindu monk, *swāmī,* and one of a world brotherhood (or holy order) of *sannyāsins.* Some are wanderers and others live in monasteries.

Sanskrit (Saṁskṛita): संस्कृत "Well-made," "refined," "perfected." The classical sacerdotal language of ancient India, considered a pure vehicle for communication with the celestial worlds. It is the primary language in which Hindu scriptures are written, including the *Vedas* and *Āgamas.* Employed today as a liturgical, literary and scholarly language, but no longer as a spoken vernacular.

santosha: सन्तोष "Contentment." See: *yama-niyama.*

sapta ṛishis: सप्तऋषि Seven inner-plane masters who help guide the *karmas* of mankind.

sārī: (Hindi, साड़ी) The traditional garment of a Hindu woman.

śāstrī: शास्त्री One who is knowledgeable in *śāstra,* or scriptures.

satguru (sadguru): सद्गुरु "True weighty one." A spiritual preceptor of the highest attainment and authority—one who has realized the ultimate Truth, Paraśiva, through *nirvikalpa samādhi*—a *jīvanmukta* able to lead others securely along the spiritual path. He is always a *sannyāsin,* an unmarried renunciate. He is recognized and revered as the embodiment of God, Sadāśiva, the source of grace and liberation.

sattva guṇa: सत्त्वगुण "Perfection of Being." The quality of goodness or purity. See: *guṇa.*

satya: सत्य "Truthfulness." See: *yama-niyama.*

śaucha: शौच "Purity." See: *yama-niyama.*

Self (Self God): God Śiva's perfection of Absolute Reality, Paraśiva—That which abides at the core of every soul. See: *Paraśiva.*

Self Realization: Direct knowing of the Self God, Paraśiva. Self Realization is known in Sanskrit as *nirvikalpa samādhi;* "enstasy without form or seed;" the ultimate spiritual attainment (also called *asamprajñata samādhi).* See: *God Realization.*

sevā: सेवा "Service," *karma yoga,* an integral part of the spiritual path, doing selfless, useful work for others, such as volunteer work at a temple, without preference or thought of reward or personal gain. *Sevā,* or Sivathondu in Tamil, is the central practice of the *charyā pāda.*

siddha: सिद्ध A "perfected one" or accomplished *yogī,* a person of great spiritual attainment or powers. See: *siddhi.*

siddhānta: सिद्धान्त "Final attainments;" "final conclusions." Ultimate understanding in any field.

siddhānta śravaṇa (or śrāvaṇa): सिद्धान्तश्रवण "Scriptural listening." See: *yama-niyama.*

siddhi: सिद्धि "Power, accomplishment; perfection." Extraordinary powers of the soul, developed through consistent meditation and deliberate, often uncomfortable and grueling *tapas,* or awakened naturally through spiritual maturity and *yogic sādhana.*

sin: Intentional transgression of divine law. Akin to the Latin *sons,* "guilty." Hinduism does not view sin as a crime against God, but as an act against *dharma*—moral order—and one's own self. Sin is an *adharmic* course of action which automatically brings negative consequences.

śishya: शिष्य "A pupil or disciple," especially one who has proven himself and been accepted by a *guru.*

Śiva: शिव The "Auspicious," "Gracious," or "Kindly one." Supreme Being of the Śaivite religion. God Śiva is All and in all, simultaneously the creator and the creation, both immanent and transcendent. As personal Deity, He is Creator, Preserver and Destroyer. He is a one Being, perhaps best understood in three perfections: Parameśvara (Primal Soul), Parāśakti (Pure Consciousness) and Paraśiva (Absolute Reality).

Śivaloka: शिवलोक "Realm of Śiva." See: *loka.*

Śivarātri: शिवरात्रि "Night of Śiva." See: *Mahāśivarātri.*

Skanda: स्कन्द "Quicksilver;" "leaping one." One of Lord Kārttikeya's oldest names, and His form as scarlet-hued warrior God.

Skanda Shashṭhī: स्कन्दषष्ठी A six-day festival in October-November celebrating Lord Kārttikeya's, or Skanda's, victory over the forces of darkness.

śloka: श्लोक A verse, phrase, proverb or hymn of praise, usually composed in a specified meter. Especially a verse of two lines, each of sixteen syllables.

Smārta: स्मार्त "Of or related to *smṛiti,*" the secondary Hindu scriptures. See: *Smārtism.*

Smārtism: स्मार्त Sect based on the secondary scriptures *(smṛiti).* The most liberal of the four major Hindu denominations, an ancient Vedic *brāhminical* tradition (ca 700 BCE) which from the 9th century onward was guided and deeply influenced by the Advaita Vedānta teachings of the reformist Adi Sankara.

soul: The real being of man, as distinguished from body, mind and emotions. The soul—known as *ātman* or *purusha*—is the sum of its two aspects, the form or body of the soul and the essence of the soul.

śraddhā: श्रद्धा "Faith; belief."

strī dharma: स्त्रीधर्म "Womanly conduct." See: *dharma.*

subconscious mind: *Saṁskāra chitta.* See: *mind (five states).*

Subramuniyaswami: சுப்பிரமுனியசுவாமி Author of this book, 162nd *satguru* (1927–2001) of the Nandinātha Sampradāya's Kailāsa Paramparā. He was recognized worldwide as one of foremost Hindu ministers of our times, contributing to the revival of Hinduism in immeasurable abundance. He was simultaneously a staunch defender of traditions, as the tried and proven ways of the past, and a fearless innovator, setting new patterns of life for contemporary humanity. For a brief biography of this remarkable seer and renaissance *guru,* see *About the Author* on page 183.

sub-subconscious mind: *Vāsanā chitta.* See: *mind (five states).*

subsuperconscious mind: *Anukāraṇa chitta.* See: *mind (five states).*

śuddha avasthā: शुद्ध अवस्था "Stage of purity." (Tamil: *avasthai.*) In Śaiva Siddhānta, the last of three stages of evolution, in which the soul is immersed in Śiva. Self Realization having been attained, the mental body is purified and thus reflects the divine soul nature, Śiva's nature, more than in the *kevala* or *sakala* state. Now the soul continues to unfold through the stages of realization, and ultimately merges back into its source, the Primal Soul. See: *avasthā, kevala avasthā, sakala avasthā.*

superconscious mind: *Kāraṇa chitta.* See: *mind (five states), mind (three phases).*

sushumṇā nāḍī: सुषुम्णानाडी "Most gracious channel." Central psychic nerve current within the spinal column. See: *kuṇḍalinī, nāḍī.*

sutala chakra: सुतल चक्र "Great abyss." Region of obsessive jealousy and retaliation.

The third *chakra* below the *mūlādhāra,* centered in the knees. Corresponds to the third astral netherworld beneath the Earth's surface, called Saṁhāta ("abandoned") or Sutala. See: *chakra, Narakaloka.*

sūtra: सूत्र "Thread." An aphoristic verse; the literary style consisting of such maxims. From 500 BCE, this style was widely adopted by Indian philosophical systems and eventually employed in works on law, grammar, medicine, poetry, crafts, etc.

svadharma: स्वधर्म "One's own way." See: *dharma.*

svādhishṭhāna: स्वाधिष्ठान "One's own base." See: *chakra.*

synonymous with *Svarloka.* See: *loka.*

swāmī: स्वामी "Lord; owner; self-possessed." He who knows or is master of himself. A respectful title for a Hindu monk, usually a *sannyāsin,* an initiated, orange-robed renunciate, dedicated wholly to religious life. As a sign of respect, the term *swāmī* is sometimes applied more broadly to include non-monastics dedicated to spiritual work.

talātala chakra: तलातल चक्र "Lower region." The fourth *chakra* below the *mūlādhāra,* centered in the calves. Region of chronic mental confusion and unreasonable stubbornness. Corresponds to the fourth astral netherworld beneath the Earth's surface, called Tāmisra ("darkness") or Talātala. This state of consciousness is born of the sole motivation of self-preservation. See: *chakra, Narakaloka.*

tamas(ic): तमस् "Force of inertia." See: *guṇa.*

Tamil: தமிழ் The ancient Dravidian language of the Tamils, a Caucasoid people of South India and Northern Sri Lanka, who have now migrated throughout the world. The official language of the state of Tamil Nadu, India, spoken by 60 million people.

tantra: तन्त्र "Loom, methodology." 1) Most generally, a synonym for *śāstra,* "scripture." 2) A synonym for the Āgamic texts, especially those of the Śākta faith, a class of Hindu scripture providing detailed instruction on all aspects of religion, mystic knowledge and science. The *tantras* are also associated with the Śaiva tradition. 3) A specific method, technique or spiritual practice within the Śaiva and Śākta traditions. 4) Disciplines and techniques with a strong emphasis on worship of the feminine force, often involving sexual encounters, with the purported goal of transformation and union with the Divine.

tapas: तपस् "Heat, fire; ardor." Purificatory spiritual disciplines, severe austerity, penance and sacrifice. The endurance of pain, suffering, through the performance of extreme penance, religious austerity and mortification.

tapasvin: तपस्विन् One who performs *tapas* or is in the state of *tapas.* See: *tapas.*

That: When capitalized, this simple demonstrative refers uniquely to the Ultimate, Indescribable or Nameless Absolute. The Self God, Paraśiva.

Third World: Śivaloka, "realm of Śiva," or Kāraṇaloka. The spiritual realm or causal plane of existence wherein Mahādevas and highly evolved souls live in their own self-effulgent forms. See: *loka, three worlds.*

three worlds: The three worlds of existence, *triloka,* are the primary hierarchical divisions of the cosmos. 1) Bhūloka: "Earth world," the physical plane. 2) Antarloka: "Inner or in-between world," the subtle or astral plane. 3) Śivaloka: "World of Śiva," and of the Gods and highly evolved souls; the causal plane, also called Kāraṇaloka.

tirodhāna śakti: तिरोधानशक्ति "Concealing power." Veiling grace, or God's power to obscure the soul's divine nature. *Tirodhāna śakti* is the particular energy of Śiva that binds the three bonds of *āṇava, karma, māyā* to the soul. It is a purposeful limiting of consciousness to give the opportunity to the soul to grow and mature through experience of the world.

Tirukural: **திருக்குறள்** "Holy couplets." A treasury of Hindu ethical insight and a literary masterpiece of the Tamil language, written by Śaiva Saint Tiruvalluvar (ca 200 BCE) near present-day Chennai. One of the world's earliest ethical texts, the *Tirukural* could well be considered a bible on virtue for the human race. See: *Tiruvalluvar.*

tīrthayātrā: **तीर्थयात्रा** "Journey to a holy place." Pilgrimage. See: *pilgrimage.*

Tirumantiram: **திருமந்திரம்** "Holy incantation." The Nandinātha Sampradāya's oldest Tamil scripture; written ca 200 BCE by Rishi Tirumular. It is the earliest of the *Tirumurai* texts, and a vast storehouse of esoteric *yogic* and *tantric* knowledge. It contains the mystical essence of *rāja yoga* and *siddha yoga,* and the fundamental doctrines of the 28 *Śaiva Siddhānta Āgamas,* which are the heritage of the ancient pre-historic traditions of Śaivism. As the *Āgamas* themselves are now partially lost, the 3,047-verse *Tirumantiram* is a rare source of the complete *Āgamanta* (collection of Āgamic lore). See: *Tirumular, Tirumurai.*

Tirumular: **திருமூலர்** An illustrious *siddha yogī* and *ṛishi* of the Nandinātha Sampradāya's Kailāsa Paramparā who came from the Himalayas (ca 200 BCE) to Tamil Nadu to compose the *Tirumantiram.* In this scripture he recorded the tenets of Śaivism in concise and precise verse form, based upon his own realizations and the supreme authority of the *Śaiva Āgamas* and the *Vedas.* Tirumular was a disciple of Maharishi Nandinatha. See: *Kailāsa Paramparā, Tirumantiram.*

Tirumurai: **திருமுறை** "Holy book." A twelve-book collection of hymns and writings of South Indian Śaivite saints, compiled by Saint Nambiyandar Nambi (ca 1000). The first seven books are known as *Devarams.*

Tiruvalluvar: **திருவள்ளுவர்** "Holy weaver." Tamil weaver and householder saint (ca 200 BCE) who wrote the classic Śaivite ethical scripture Tirukural. He lived with his wife Vasuki, famed for her remarkable loyalty and virtues, near modern-day Chennai. See: *Tirukural.*

tithe (tithing): The spiritual discipline, often a *vrata,* of giving one tenth of one's gainful and gifted income to a religious organization of one's choice, thus sustaining spiritual education and upliftment on earth. The Sanskrit equivalent is *daśamāṁśa,* called *makimai* in the Tamil tradition.

Truth: When capitalized, ultimate knowing which is unchanging. Lower case (truth): honesty, integrity; virtue.

upadeśa: **उपदेश** "Advice; religious instruction." Often given in question-and-answer form from *guru* to disciple. The *satguru's* spiritual discourses.

Upanishad: **उपनिषद्** "Sitting near devotedly." The fourth and final portion of the *Vedas,* expounding the secret, philosophical meaning of the Vedic hymns. The *Upanishads* are a collection of profound texts which are the source of Vedānta and have dominated Indian thought for thousands of years. They are philosophical chronicles of *ṛishis* expounding the nature of God, soul and cosmos, exquisite renderings of the deepest Hindu thought. The number of *Upanishads* is given as 108.

Vaishṇava: वैष्णव Of or relating to Vishṇu; same as Vaishṇavite. A follower of Lord Vishṇu or His incarnations. See: *Vaishṇavism, Vishṇu.*

Vaishṇavism (Vaishṇava): वैष्णव One of the four major religions, or denominations of Hinduism, representing roughly half of the world's one billion Hindus. It gravitates around the worship of Lord Vishṇu as Personal God, His incarnations and their consorts. Vaishṇavism stresses the personal aspect of God over the impersonal, and *bhakti* (devotion) as the true path to salvation.

Vaishṇavite: Of or relating to Vishṇu; same as Vaishṇava. A follower of Vishṇu or His incarnations. See: *Vaishṇavism, Vishnu.*

vāsanā: वासना "Abode." Subconscious inclinations. From *vās,* "dwelling, residue, remainder." The subliminal inclinations and habit patterns which, as driving forces, color and motivate one's attitudes and future actions.

vāsanā daha tantra: वासनादहतन्त्र "Purification of the subconscious by fire." *Daha* means burning, *tantra* is a method, and *vāsanās* are deep-seated subconscious traits or tendencies that shape one's attitudes and motivations. *Vāsanās* can be ether positive or negative. One of the best methods for resolving difficulties in life, of dissolving troublesome *vāsanās,* the *vāsanā daha tantra* is the practice of burning confessions, or even long letters to loved ones or acquaintances, describing pains, expressing confusions and registering grievances and long-felt hurts. Also called spiritual journaling, writing down problems and burning them in any ordinary fire brings them from the subconscious into the external mind, releasing the supressed emotion as the fire consumes the paper. This is a magical healing process. —***mahā vāsanā daha tantra:*** The special sādhana of looking back over and writing about the various aspects of one's life in order to clear all accumulated subconscious burdens, burning the papers as done in the periodic vāsana daha tantra. Ten pages are to be written about each year. Other aspects of this tantra include writing about people one has known (people check), all sexual experiences (sex check).

Veda: वेद् "Wisdom." Sagely revelations which comprise Hinduism's most authoritative scripture. They, along with the *Āgamas,* are *śruti,* that which is "heard." The *Vedas* are a body of dozens of holy texts known collectively as the *Veda,* or as the four *Vedas: Ṛig, Yajur, Sāma* and *Atharva.* In all they include over 100,000 verses, as well as additional prose. The knowledge imparted by the *Vedas* ranges from earthy devotion to high philosophy.

Vedānta: वेदान्त "Ultimate wisdom" or "final conclusions of the *Vedas.*" Vedānta is the system of thought embodied in the *Upanishads* (ca 1500-600 BCE), which give forth the ultimate conclusions of the *Vedas.* Through history there developed numerous Vedānta schools, ranging from pure dualism to absolute monism.

Vedic-Āgamic: Simultaneously drawing from and complying with both of Hinduism's revealed scriptures *(śruti), Vedas* and *Āgamas,* which represent two complimentary, intertwining streams of history and tradition.

vegetarian: *Śakāhāra.* Of a diet which excludes meat, fish, fowl and eggs. Vegetarianism is a principle of health and environmental ethics that has been a keystone of Indian life for thousands of years. Vegetarian foods include grains, fruits, vegetables, legumes and dairy products. Natural, fresh foods, locally grown, without insecticides or chemical fertilizers, are preferred. The following foods are minimized: frozen and canned foods, highly processed foods, such as white rice, white sugar and white flour; and "junk" foods and beverages (those with abundant chemical additives, such as artificial sweeteners, colorings, flavorings and preservatives, or prepared with unwholesome ingredients).

veiling grace: *Tirobhāva śakti.* The divine power that limits the soul's perception by binding or attaching the soul to the bonds of *āṇava, karma,* and *māyā*— enabling it to grow and evolve as an individual being.

vibhūti: विभूति "Resplendent, powerful." Holy ash, prepared by burning cow dung along with other precious substances, milk, *ghee,* honey, etc. It symbolizes purity and is one of the main sacraments given at *pūjā* in all Śaivite temples and shrines.

Vishṇu: विष्णु "All-pervasive." Supreme Deity of the Vaishṇavite religion. God as personal Lord and Creator, the All-Loving Divine Personality, who periodically incarnates and lives a fully human life to reestablish *dharma* whenever necessary. In Śaivism, Vishṇu is Śiva's aspect as Preserver. See: *Vaishṇavism.*

viśuddha chakra: विशुद्धचक्र "Wheel of purity." The fifth *chakra.* Center of divine love. See: *chakra.*

Viśvaguru: विश्वगुरु "World as teacher." The playful personification of the world as the *guru* of those with no *guru,* headmaster of the school of hard knocks, where students are left to their own devices and learn by their own mistakes rather than by following a traditional teacher.

vitala chakra: वितल चक्र "Region of negation." Region of raging anger and viciousness. The second *chakra* below the *mūlādhāra,* centered in the thighs. Corresponds to the second astral netherworld beneath the earth's surface, called Avīchi ("joyless") or Vitala. See: *chakra, Narakaloka.*

vivāha: विवाह "Marriage." See: *saṁskāras.*

vrata: व्रत "Vow, religious oath." Often a vow to perform certain disciplines, such as penance, fasting, specific *mantra* repetitions, worship or meditation.

yajña: यज्ञ "Worship; sacrifice." One of the most central Hindu concepts—sacrifice and surrender through acts of worship, inner and outer. 1) Primarily, yajña is a form of ritual worship especially prevalent in Vedic times, in which oblations—*ghee,* grains, spices and exotic woods—are offered into a fire according to scriptural injunctions while special *mantras* are chanted. The element fire, *Agni,* is revered as the divine messenger who carries offerings and prayers to the Gods. *Yajña* requires four components, none of which may be omitted: *dravya,* sacrificial substances; *tyāga,* the spirit of sacrificing all to God; *devatā,* the celestial beings who receive the sacrifice; and *mantra,* the empowering word or chant. 2) *Manushya yajña* or often *simply yajña,* "homage to men," is feeding guests and the poor, the homeless and the student. *Manushya yajña* includes all acts of philanthropy, such as tithing and charity. In Sri Lanka, *yajña* (Tamil, *yagam*) also refers to large, ceremonious mass feedings.

yama-niyama: यम नियम The first two of the eight limbs of *rāja yoga,* constituting Hinduism's fundamental ethical codes, the *yamas* and *niyamas* are the essential foundation for all spiritual progress. Here are the ten traditional *yamas* and ten *niyamas.* —***yamas:*** 1) ***ahiṁsā:*** "Noninjury." Not harming others by thought, word, or deed. 2) ***satya:*** "Truthfulness." Refraining from lying and betraying promises. 3) ***asteya:*** "Nonstealing." Neither stealing, nor coveting nor entering into debt. 4) ***brahmacharya:*** "Divine conduct." Controlling lust by remaining celibate when single, leading to faithfulness in marriage. 5) ***kshamā:*** "Patience." Restraining intolerance with people and impatience with circumstances. 6) ***dhṛiti:*** "Steadfastness." Overcoming nonperseverance, fear, indecision and changeableness. 7) ***dayā:*** "Compassion." Conquering callous, cruel and insensitive feelings toward all beings. 8) ***ārjava:*** "Honesty, straightforwardness." Renouncing deception and wrongdoing. 9) ***mitāhāra:*** "Moderate appetite." Neither eating too much nor consuming meat, fish, fowl or eggs. 10) ***śaucha:*** "Purity." Avoiding impurity in body, mind and speech. —***niyamas:*** 1) ***hrī:*** "Remorse." Being modest and showing shame for misdeeds. 2) ***santosha:*** "Contentment." Seeking joy and serenity in life. 3) ***dāna:*** "Giving." Tithing and giving generously without thought of reward. 4) ***āstikya:*** "Faith." Believing firmly in God, Gods, *guru* and the path to enlightenment. 5) **Īśvarapūjana:** "Worship of the Lord." The cultivation of devotion through daily worship and meditation. 6) ***siddhānta śravaṇa:*** "Scriptural audition." Studying the teachings and listening to the wise of one's lineage. 7) ***mati:*** "Cognition." Developing a spiritual will and intellect with the *guru's* guidance. 8) ***vrata:*** "Sacred vows." Fulfilling religious vows, rules and observances faithfully. 9) ***japa:*** "Recitation." Chanting *mantras* daily. 10) ***tapas:*** "Austerity." Performing *sādhana,* penance, *tapas* and sacrifice. Patanjali lists the *yamas* as: *ahiṁsā, satya, asteya, brahmacharya* and *aparigraha* (noncovetousness); and the *niyamas* as: *śaucha, santosha, tapas, svādhyāya* (self-reflection, private scriptural study) and Īśvarapraṇidhāna (worship). See: *ashṭaṅga yoga.*

yoga: योग "Union." From *yuj,* "to yoke, harness, unite." The philosophy, process, disciplines and practices whose purpose is the yoking of individual consciousness with transcendent or divine consciousness. See: *ashṭaṅga yoga.*

yoga pāda: योगपाद The third of the successive stages in spiritual unfoldment in Śaiva Siddhānta, wherein the goal is Self Realization. See: *pāda.*

Yogaswami (Yogaswāmī): யோகசுவாமி "Master of *yoga.*" Sri Lanka's most renowned contemporary spiritual master (1872–1964), a Sivajñāni and Nātha *siddhar* revered by both Hindus and Buddhists. He was trained by Satguru Chellappaswami, from whom he received *guru dīkshā.* Sage Yogaswami was the *satguru* of Sivaya Subramuniyaswami. Yogaswami conveyed his teachings songs called *Natchintanai,* "good thoughts." See: *Kailāsa Paramparā.*

yogī: योगी One who practices *yoga.*

yoginī: योगिनी Feminine counterpart of *yogī.*

yuga: युग "Eon," "age." One of four ages which chart the duration of the world according to Hindu thought: Satya (or Kṛita), Tretā, Dvāpara and Kali. In the first period, *dharma* reigns supreme, but as the ages revolve, virtue diminishes and ignorance and injustice increases. At the end of the Kali Yuga, in which we are now, the cycle begins again with a new Satya Yuga.

Sanskrit Pronunciation

Ucchāraṇam Saṁskṛita उच्चारणम् संस्कृत

VOWELS

Vowels marked like ā are sounded twice as long as short vowels. The four dipthongs, *e, ai, o, au,* are always sounded long, but never marked as such.

अ a as in about
आ ा ā ...tar, father
इ ि i ...fill, lily
ई ी ī ...machine
उ ु u ...full, bush
ऊ ू ū ...allude
ऋ ृ ṛi ...merrily
ॠ ॄ ṛī ...marine
ऌ lṛi ...revelry
ए े e ...prey
ऐ ै ai ...aisle
ओ ो o ...go, stone
औ ौ au ...Haus

GUTTURAL CONSONANTS

Sounded in the throat.

क् k ...kite, seek
ख् kh ...inkhorn
ग् g ...gamble
घ् gh ...loghouse
ङ् ṅ ...sing

PALATAL CONSONANTS

Sounded at the roof of the mouth.

च् ch ...church
छ् çh ...much harm
ज् j ...jump
झ् jh ...hedgehog
ञ् ñ ...hinge

CEREBRAL CONSONANTS

Tongue turned up and back against the roof of the mouth. (Also known as retroflex.)

ट् ṭ ...true
ठ् ṭh ...nuthook
ड् ḍ ...drum
ढ् ḍh ...redhaired
ण् ṇ ...none

DENTAL CONSONANTS

Sounded with the tip of the tongue at the back of the upper front teeth.

त् t ...tub
थ् th ...anthill
द् d ...dot
ध् dh ...adhere
न् n ...not

LABIAL CONSONANTS

Sounded at the lips.

प् p ...pot
फ् ph ...path
ब् b ...bear
भ् bh ...abhor
म् m ...map

SEMIVOWELS

य् y ...yet (palatal)
र् ॅ r ...road (cereb.)
ल् l ...lull (dental)
व् v ...voice (labial), but more like w when following a consonant, as in *swāmī.*
ह् h ...hear (guttural)

SIBILANTS

श् ś ...sure (palatal)
ष् sh ...shut (cerebral)
स् s ...saint (dental)

ANUSVĀRA

The dot over Devanāgarī letters represents the nasal of the type of letter it precedes; e.g.: अंग = aṅga. It is transliterated as ṁ or as the actual nasal (ṅ, ñ, n, ṇ, m). At the end of words it is sometimes म् (m).

VISĀRGA (:) **ḥ**

Pronounced like *huh* (with a short, stopping sound), or *hih,* after i, ī and e.

ASPIRATES

The h following a consonant indicates aspiration, the addition of air, as in nātha or bhakti. Thus, th should not be confused with th in the word then.

Special Characters

ज्ञ् jñ ...a nasalized sound, like gya or jya.
क्ष् = क्+ ष् ksh

CONVENTIONS

1. As a rule, the root forms of Sanskṛit words are used (without case endings).
2. च्छ is transliterated as cçh, and च्च as cch.
3. Geographical and personal names (e.g., *Hardwar),* are generally marked with diacriticals only as main lexicon entries.
4. Diacritical marks are not used for Tamil words.

Index

Anukramaṇikā अनुक्रमणिका

E

F

Face: loss of, 62
Faith: See *Āstikya*
Faithfulness: in marriage, 17, 20, 124
Family: daily meetings of, xiii; destroyed by adultery, 22; mutual respect in, 2; society and, 8; worshiping together, 94. See also *Children; Home; Marriage; Parenting*
Fasting: for health, 46
Faults: wise handling of, 7
Favors: indebtedness and, 40
Fear: *atala chakra,* 115; lower consciousness, 45; meat-eating and, 48; overcoming, 29; and untruthfulness, 5; willpower drained by, 115, 117
Feedings: mass, 78
Feelings: *karma* created by, 35
Fickleness: flexibility vs., 30
Fish: not consuming, 45, 47-48. See *Vegetarianism*
Flexibility: fickleness vs., 30
Food: offering to God, 97; purity in, 51-52, 55. See also *Diet*
Food-blessing *mantra:* excerpt, 67
Forbearance: monastics &, 27
Forgiveness: compassion and, 33; seeking, 58, 62
Fowl: not consuming, 45, 47-48. See *Vegetarianism*
Friends: See *Companions*
Fulfillment: giving as, 73-74; wife's, 77
Fundamentalism: violence and, 2

G

Gambling: "Gambler's Lament" (Vedic quote), 14; nonparticipation in, 13-14
Gandhi, Mahatma: celibacy of, 20, 122
Gaṇeśa: functions of, 123
Giving: *karmic* law, 73, 75; to *satguru,* 77; for tax deductions, 74; gifts of time, 75-76; wives', 76-77. See also *Dāna*
Goals: contentment and, 68
God and Gods: faith in, 85; living in God's house, 96-98; reality of, 96; stage of, see *Arul pada;* and *tapas,* 132; vows to, 119, 122-124; worship of, 94-95, 99. See also *God Śiva; Worship*
God Realization: See *Samādhi*
God Śiva: guests as, 74; seeing in all, 98. See also *God and Gods*
Grace: concealing (veiling), 74, 86, 88; descent of, 88; *guru's,* 57, 109-111; invoking, 95; revealing, 88; stage of, see *Arul pada;* and worship, 94
Guests: treated as God, 74, 96. See also *Hospitality*
Guilt: instinctive quality, 60. See also *Remorse*
Guru: approaching, 103, 128; and austerity, 135; books written by, 104; choosing wisely, 103, 111, 128; and cognition, 109; faith in, 85; first encounter, 102, 107, 120; guidance of, 109-111, 120, 127; grace of, 57, 109-111; honesty with, 7, 39, 127-128; initiation by, 120-121, 127-128; inner communication, 114; and *japa/mantra,* 102, 127; mitigating *karmas,* 12; one step/nine steps, 104; role of, 7-8; and *sādhana,* 29; and *sushumṇā nāḍīs,* 105-106, 110; television as, 113; and vows, 119, 122-124; world as, 12. See also *Initiation; Sampradāya; Satguru*

H

Habits: replacing unwanted, 54
Hamlet: quote from, 37
Hardship: See *Adversity*
Haṭha Yoga Pradīpikā: *yamas* and *niyamas* in, xiii
Healing: from misdeeds, 62
Health: diet and, 43-48; moderation and, 43; treasure, 68
Hinduism: conglomerate, 63; ethical code of, vii, xiii; importance of ahiṁsā, 34; liberal sects, 96; philosophical basis for noninjury, 1-2; based on *Vedas,* 106
Home: extension of temple, 95; God's

Scriptural Citations

The following are the scriptures and sourcebooks from which quotations in Yoga's Forgotten Foundation ***were drawn***

Invocation from the *Iśa Upanishad, Śukla Yajur Veda* (cited on p. 67).
Ṛig Veda 10.34 (cited on p. 14); *The Vedic Experience* (p. 50), Panikkar, Raimond (Delhi, Motilal Banarsidass, 1989).
Śāndilya Upanishad (cited on p. 29); *Thirty Minor Upanishads, Including the Yoga Upanishads* (p. 173-174), K. Narayanasvami Aiyar (Oklahoma, Santarasa Publications, 1980).
Tirukural, by Saint Tiruvalluvar (cited on p. 6, 13, 30, 135); *Weaver's Wisdom, Ancient Precepts for a Perfect Life*, Sivaya Subramuniyaswami (Hawaii, Himalayan Academy, 1999).
Tirumantiram (cited on p. xix); *Tirumantiram, Holy Uterances of Saint Tirumular*, Dr. B. Natarajan et al. (Hawaii, Saiva Siddhanta Church, 1982).

Colophon

Antyavachanam अन्त्यवदानम्

YOGA'S FORGOTTEN FOUNDATION WAS DESIGNED AND ILLUSTRATED BY THE *ĀCHĀRYAS* AND *SWĀMĪS* OF THE ŚAIVA SIDDHĀNTA YOGA ORDER AT KAUAI AADHEENAM, KAUAI'S Hindu Monastery on Hawaii's Garden Island. It was produced on Macintosh G4 computers using Adobe InDesign 2, Adobe Photoshop 7 and Adobe Illustrator 10. The text is set in Adobe's Minion family of fonts (with diacritical marks added using Fontographer): 11.5-point regular on 13.5-point linespacing for the body of the book and 8.25 on 9.75 for the glossary and index. Sanskrit and Tamil fonts are by Ecological Linguistics and Srikrishna Patil. Printing production was supervised by Tiru A. Sothinathan of Uma Publications in Kuala Lumpur, with printing by four-color offset press executed at Sampoorna Printers Sdn. Bhd. on 85 gsm coated art paper. ¶The cover art is a watercolor by Tiru S. Rajam, 84, of Chennai, India. The painting on the half-title page is by the same artist. The oil portrait of Gurudeva on the back cover was a gift by renowned artist Sri Indra Sharma during a sojourn on Kauai in 1997. The watercolor paintings that initiate each chapter are the work of Tiru A. Manivelu, 62. The background patterns adorning the title pages were created by the monastics using Adobe Photoshop. The book's index was created by Tirumati Chamundi Sabanathan of Santa Rosa, California, using Sonar Bookends. Sanskrit translation of the chapter titles was provided by Dr. Sarasvati Mohan of Campbell, California. ¶We know that Gurudeva is smiling down upon this book from the inner planes, pleased with its production, happy that his original vision has been fulfilled, lending his blessings to all those who read his words and strive to apply this earthy wisdom to their daily life. Aum.

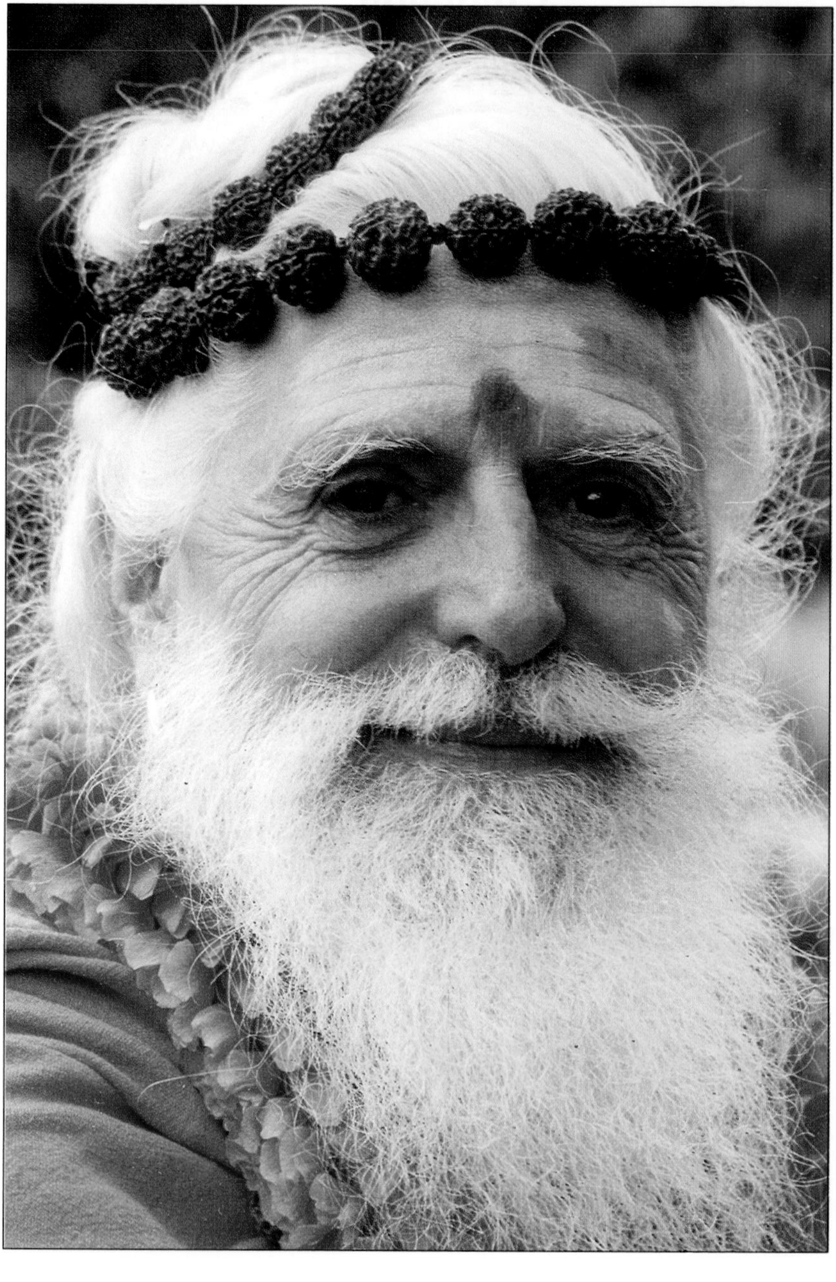

About the Author

ONCE IN A GREAT WHILE ON THIS EARTH THERE ARISES A SOUL WHO, BY LIVING HIS TRADITION RIGHTLY AND WHOLLY, PERFECTS HIS PATH AND A BECOMES A LIGHT TO THE WORLD. Satguru Sivaya Subramuniyaswami (1927-2001) was such a being, a shining example of awakening and wisdom, a leader recognized worldwide as one of Hinduism's foremost ministers. ¶As a youth, he was trained in classical Eastern and Western dance and in the disciplines of *yoga.* Becoming the premier danseur of the San Francisco Ballet by age 19, he renounced the world at the height of his career and traveled to India and Sri Lanka in quest of Absolute Truth. In the caves of Jalani in 1949, he fasted and meditated until he burst into enlightenment. Soon thereafter, he met his *satguru,* Sage Yogaswami, who gave him the name *Subramuniya,* initiated him into the holy orders of *sannyāsa* and ordained him into his lineage with a tremendous slap on the back, saying, "This sound will be heard in America! Now go 'round the world and roar like a lion. You will build palaces (temples) and feed thousands." While in Sri Lanka, he founded Saiva Siddhanta Church, the world's first Hindu church, now active in many nations. In late 1949 he sailed back to America and embarked on seven years of ardent, solitary *yoga* and meditation which brought forth faculties of clairvoyance and clairaudience, culminating in *Cognizantability,* a collection of profound aphorisms and commentary on the states of mind and esoteric laws of life. In 1957, Subramuniyaswami, affectionately known as Gurudeva, founded Himalayan Academy and opened America's first Hindu temple, in San Francisco. He formed his monastic order in 1960. In Switzerland, 1968, he revealed Shūm, a mystical language of meditation that names and maps inner areas of consciousness. From 1967 to 1983 he led fourteen Innersearch pilgrimages, guiding hundreds of devotees to the world's sacred temples and illumined sages. In 1970 Gurudeva established his world headquarters and monastery-temple on Kauai, northernmost of the Hawaiian Islands. Beginning in the 1970s and continuing to 2001, he gave blessings to dozens of groups to build temples in North America, Australia, New Zealand, Europe and elsewhere, gifting Deity images, usually of Lord Gaṇeśa, to 36 temples to begin the worship. Over the years, he personally guided groups of trustees through each stage of temple development. He thus authenticated and legitimized the establishment of the temple as essential to any Hindu community. His relentless drive to establish Hindu worship in the West was based on his revelatory mystic visions of the Gods not as symbolic depictions but as real beings who guide and protect mankind, with whom we can commune most effectively through consecrated temples. ¶In 1973, after establishing Kadavul Temple, he clairvoyantly read from inner-plane libraries to bring forth *Lemurian Scrolls* and other esoteric writings to guide his monastic order and revive the centrality of celibacy and sexual transmutation. In 1975, following a powerful vision of Lord Śiva, he conceived the San Marga Iraivan Temple on Kauai as the first all-granite temple established outside of India. In 1977 he intensified requirements for his Western devotees to sever all prior religious, philosophical loyalties, legalize their Hindu name and formally enter Hinduism through the name-giving rite. In 1979 he published *Holy Orders of Sannyāsa,* defining the ideals, vows and aspirations of Hindu monasticism with unprecedented clarity. That same year, he began publishing HINDUISM TODAY magazine. His international Hindu renaissance tours in the early '80s revealed that Hindus were not globally connected or organized. Those in India knew little of their brothers and sisters in South America. Those in Fiji had no knowledge of Hindus in Europe or Mauritius. Seeing this need, Gurudeva focused his journal on uniting all Hindus, regardless of nationality or sect, and inspiring and educating seekers everywhere. Also in 1979, he produced the first edition of his Hindu catechism, later to become *Dancing with Śiva.* ¶His travels in the 1980s brought him face to face with hundreds of thousands of Hindus, most notably in Sri Lanka, India, Malaysia and Mauritius, to whom he spread a powerful message of courage and was instrumental in regenerating pride of heritage. In the early '80s he established the antiquity and legitimacy of monistic Śaiva Siddhānta at international conferences among pundits who had insisted that Siddhānta is solely pluralistic. In 1985 Gurudeva adopted Apple's Macintosh-based publishing technology to supercharge his prolific outreach through scriptures, books, pamphlets, art, lessons and later through CDs and the world's foremost Hindu websites. ¶In 1986 he founded a branch monastery in Mauritius, whose government had invited him there to revive a languishing Hindu faith. That same year, New Delhi's World Religious Parliament named him one of five modern-day Jagadāchāryas, world teachers, for his international efforts in promoting a Hindu renaissance. Also in 1986 he created Pañcha Gaṇapati, a five-day

Hindu festival celebrated around the time of Christmas. In 1987 he published *God's Money* to explain tithing and how it is practiced by members of his Hindu church. The year 1989 saw the culmination of numerous books and pamphlets that later became part of the Master Course trilogy. In 1990 in Bangalore, he ceremoniously chipped the first stone of Iraivan temple and established a small village where craftsmen and their families could live and carve this architectural gem by hand over the next fifteen years. In 1991 he produced the *Nandinātha Sūtras*, 365 aphorisms outlining the entire gamut of virtuous Hindu living. In 1994 Gurudeva founded Hindu Heritage Endowment, now a multi-million-dollar public service trust that establishes and maintains permanent sources of income for Hindu institutions worldwide. In 1995 he published the final edition of *Śaiva Dharma Śāstras*, drawing on aspects of the American church system to make his organization socially viable and structurally effective. Therein he finalized patterns for the future, including the extended family structure for his missions, and designated as his successors three of his senior monastics: Acharya Veylanswami, followed by Acharya Palaniswami and then Acharya Ceyonswami. ¶From 1977 to 2001 Gurudeva nurtured a staunchly Hindu, highly disciplined, global fellowship of family initiates, monastics and students, training them to follow the *sādhana mārga*, the path of *yogic* striving and personal transformation, and to assist him in his global mission. With this competent team and a sophisticated infrastructure, his Church nurtures its membership and local missions on five continents and serves, personally and through publications and the Internet, the community of Hindus of all sects. It furthers the dual mission of Hindu solidarity and monistic Śaiva Siddhānta, vowing to protect, preserve and promote the Śaivite Hindu religion as expressed through three pillars: temples, *satgurus* and scripture. The recognized hereditary *guru* of 2.5 million Sri Lankan Hindus, Gurudeva proclaimed his Church a Jaffna-Tamil-based organization which branched out from the Sri Subramuniya Ashram in Alaveddy to meet the needs of the growing Hindu diaspora of this century. It gently oversees some 40 temples worldwide. Missionaries and teachers within the family membership provide counseling and classes in Śaivism for children, youth and adults. Gurudeva's numerous books present his unique and practical insights on Hindu metaphysics, mysticism, culture, philosophy and *yoga*. His *Śaivite Hindu Religion* children's course is taught in many temples and homes, preserving the teachings in five languages for thousands of youths. ¶In 1995, in Delhi, the World Religious Parliament bestowed on him the title Dharmachakra for his remarkable publications. The Global Forum of Spiritual and Parliamentary Leaders for Human Survival chose him as a Hindu representative at its momentus conferences. Thus, at Oxford in 1988, Moscow in 1990 and Rio de Janeiro in 1992, he joined religious, political and scientific leaders from all countries to discuss the future of human life on this planet. At Chicago's historic centenary Parliament of the World's Religions in September, 1993, he was elected one of three Hindus to the Presidents' Assembly, a core group of 25 men and women voicing the needs of world faiths. Especially in the early '90s he campaigned for fair treatment of temple priests, namely the same respect enjoyed by the clergy of other religions. From 1996 onward, Gurudeva was a key member of Vision Kauai 2020, a group of inspirers (including the Mayor, county council, business and education leaders) that meets to fashion the island's future based on spiritual values. In 1997 he responded to President Clinton's call for religious opinions on the ethics of human cloning. That same year, he spearheaded the 125th anniversary of Satguru Yogaswami and his golden icon's pilgrimage around the world, ending in Sri Lanka. During these final years he worked daily in the morning hours in refining the Shūm language as his supreme gift to his monastic order. ¶In 1998 Gurudeva began an ardent campaign for the right of children to not be beaten by their parents or their teachers, helping parents raise children with love through Positive Discipline classes taught by his family devotees as their primary community service. In 1999 he traveled to Mauritius to publicly inaugurate his Spiritual Park as a gift to the island nation. In 2000 he published *How to Become a Hindu,* showing the way for seekers to formally enter the faith, refuting the dogma that "You must be born a Hindu to be a Hindu." On August 25, 2000, he received the prestigious United Nations U Thant Peace Award in New York (previously bestowed on the Dalai Lama, Nelson Mandela, Mikhail Gorbachev, Pope John Paul II and Mother Teresa). He addressed 1,200 spiritual leaders gathered for the UN Millennium Peace Summit, with the message, "For peace in the world, stop the war in the home." Upon his return to Kauai, 350 citizens and county and state officials gathered to herald his accomplishments on the island and beyond. Governor Benjamin Cayetano wrote: "I am especially grateful for your efforts to promote moral and spiritual values in Hawaii. May our people forever embrace the message of peace you have so eloquently supported in your gracious wisdom." In November, 2000, Gurudeva launched Hindu Press International (HPI), a HINDUISM TODAY daily news summary for breaking news sent free via e-mail and posted on the web. In 1999, 2000 and 2001 he conducted three Innersearch journeys, taking devotees to Alaska, the Caribbean and Northern Europe, consecrating new temples in Alaska, Trinidad and Denmark. In 2001 he completed his golden legacy, the 3,000-page Master Course trilogy of *Dancing, Living* and *Merging with Śiva*—peerless volumes of daily lessons on Hindu philosophy, culture and *yoga,* respectively. ¶For fifty years, Subramuniyaswami taught Hinduism to Hindus and seekers from all faiths. Known as one of the strictest *gurus* in the world, he was the 162nd successor of the Nandinātha Kailāsa lineage and *satguru* of Kauai Aadheenam, his 458-acre temple-monastery complex on the Garden Island of Kauai. From this verdant Polynesian *aśrama* on a river bank near the foot of an extinct volcano, his monastics continue to promote the *dharma* together through Saiva Siddhanta Church, Himalayan Academy and Hindu Heritage Endowment, perpetuating the mission given to Gurudeva by his *satguru.* ¶Gurudeva departed from this world as courageously as he had lived in it. Learning on October 9, 2001, that he had advanced, metastacized intestinal cancer, confirmed by a host of specialists in three states, all concurring that even the most aggressive treatment regimens would not prove effective, he declined any treatment beyond palliative measures and decided to follow the Indian yogic practice, called *prāyopaveśa* in Sanskrit scripture, to abstain from nourishment and take water only from that day on. He left his body peacefully on the 32nd day of his self-declared fast, at 11:54 pm on Monday, Chitra *nakshatra,* November 12, 2001, surrounded by his twenty-three monastics. Gurudeva consoled them, "Don't be sad. When I am gone from this world, I will be working with you on the inside twenty-four hours a day." The rock-solid foundation for the continuance of his work is Kauai Aadheenam and its resident Saiva Siddhanta Yoga Order. This group of twelve initiated *swāmīs* with lifetime vows and nine *brahmachārīs,* celibate monks, come from six countries and include both men born into the Hindu religion and those who converted or adopted Hinduism—Asians and Westerners—made strong by decades of Gurudeva's loving but strict personal guidance and insistence on

110 percent performance. In the first weeks of his fast, Gurudeva seamlessly transferred his duties and responsibilities to his chosen successor, Satguru Bodhinatha Veylanswami, 59, a disciple for 37 years, declaring, "Bodhinatha is the new *satguru* now." Ever concerned for others, even on his deathbed, just days before his Great Union, he whispered in assurance, "Everything that is happening is good. Everything that is happening is meant to be." He asked devotees worldwide to carry his work and institutions forward with unstinting vigor, to keep one another strong on the spiritual path, to live in harmony and to work diligently on their personal spiritual *sādhanas.* "You are all over-qualified to carry on." ¶When notified of Gurudeva's passing, Sita Ram Goel, one of India's most influential Hindu writers and thinkers, wrote, "He has done great work for Hinduism, and the recent reawakening of the Hindu mind carries his stamp." Ma Yoga Shakti, renowned *yoga* teacher, said, "For more than five decades, Subramuniyaswami, a highly enlightened soul of the West—a Hanuman of today, a reincarnation of Śiva Himself—has watered the roots of Hinduism with great zeal, faith, enthusiasm and whole-heartedness." Sri Shivarudra Balayogi Maharaj of India said, "By his life and by his teaching, Satguru Sivaya Subramuniyaswami has helped make Hinduism an even greater gift to humanity." From Jaffna, president of Sivathondan Nilayam Arunasalam Sellathurai Swamigal wrote: "The life, mission and mandate of His Holiness Sivaya Subramuniyaswami form an epic chapter in his unending spiritual quest leading him to the founding of the Saiva Siddhanta Church and a monastic order in Hawaii—a magnificent task! This will ever remain a monument to his spiritual fervor, proclaiming worldwide, East and West, in trumpet tones that Swamigal was a trailblazer of Lord Śiva's choice to glorify the spiritual heritage and the essence of Śaiva Siddhānta." ¶Gurudeva's life was one of extraordinary accomplishments on so many levels; but his greatest *siddhi,* to which thousands of devotees will testify, was his incredible power to inspire others toward God, to change their lives in ways that are otherwise impossible, to be a light on their path, a mother and father and friend to all who drew near. Gurudeva lived so profoundly at the center of himself, so close to the core of being, the heart of Divinity, that everyone he met felt close to him. He personified the pure, blissful soul nature they sought and sensed as the center of themselves.

Milestones of His 52-Year Ministry

Enumerating a Spiritual Master's Many Gifts to Mankind

Empowered by his Self Realization, his ordination as a *satguru* and the blessings of Gods and *devas*, Gurudeva contributed to the revival of Hinduism in immeasurable abundance. He was simultaneously a staunch defender of traditions, as the proven ways of the past, and a fearless innovator, rivaling the *ṛishis* of Vedic times in instilling fresh understanding and setting new patterns of life for contemporary humanity. Here is a partial list of his trail-blazing mission and accomplishments.

SPIRITUAL TEACHINGS

- Bringing seekers new meaning to life through *The Master Course* as a path of self-transformation through *sādhana*, a self-initiated journey to bravely, cheerfully face the *karma* one has created in the past.
- Pioneering the language *Shūm* in 1968 to enhance seekers' *yogic* efforts and vigorously developing it from 1995 to 2001, as his choicest inner gift to his monastics.
- Bringing the Gods "out of exile" by explaining and writing about the mysteries of temple worship and the three worlds of existence from his own experience.
- Unfolding theological summations for a religion in renaissance, such as "Four Facts of Hinduism," "Nine Beliefs," "Hinduism's Code of Conduct," the 365 *Nandinatha Sūtras*, and a Hindu catechism and creed.
- Bringing forth *Lemurian Scrolls* and other esoteric writings from inner-plane libraries to guide his monastic order and revive the centrality of celibacy and sexual transmutation.
- Translating and publishing Tiruvalluvar's ethical masterpiece, the *Tirukural*, in modern, lucid English.

LEADING THE HINDU RENAISSANCE

- Building Hindu pride; convincing Hindus everywhere to stand up and proclaim themselves Hindus and stop repeating equivocal slogans like, "I'm not really a Hindu. I am a universalist—a Christian, a Jew, a Muslim and a Buddhist."
- Proclaiming that Hinduism is a great, living religion, not a archeologic relic of the past as oft depicted by Western scholars—one that should be presented by Hindu writers, as he did in his peerless publications.
- Teaching Hinduism to Hindus, awakening their self-appreciation as a world community, blessed inheritors of a grand civilization and culture, indeed, the religion best suited to the new age.
- Rescuing the word *Hinduism* from its fallen status as a dirty word and restoring it to its age-old glory.
- Heralding sectarianism when the prevailing trend was bland uniformity, insisting that only if each denomination is strong and faithful to its unique traditions will Hinduism itself be strong.
- Championing the centrality of temples, legitimizing their establishment, and authenticating their purpose.

CORRECTIVE CAMPAIGNS

- Dispelling myths and misinformation about Hinduism through Hinduism Today for two decades.
- Promoting the *Vedas* and *Āgamas* as the holy bible of Hinduism, rather than the mythological *Purāṇas* and the historical *Bhagavad Gītā.*
- Establishing rational mystical explanations for Hindu practice to displace the Purāṇic "comic book" mentality.
- Reinstating *ahiṁsā,* noninjury, as the cardinal ethic of Hinduism when militants were promoting righteous retaliation, often by citing the *Bhagavad Gītā.*
- Rejecting traditional stories that glorify violence, such as many found in the *Periyapuranam.*
- Repopularizing Śiva as a God of love to be worshiped by all devotees, not a fearsome being approached only by ascetics. Assuring Hindus it is all right, in fact necessary, to have Lord Śiva in the home.
- Speaking for the purity of Hindu monasticism and against the idea of "married *swāmīs*" and mixed-gender *āśramas.*
- Campaigning against the use of illegal drugs by exposing the harmful effects and *karmic* consequences.
- Combatting unethical Christian conversion by enhancing Hindu education, exposing the devious tactics of evangelists and the immaturity of faiths that consider theirs the only true path and aggressively seek to compel others to adopt it.
- Debunking the notion that "All religions are one" and publishing a comparative summary of the major religions of the world, side by side with prominent secular philosophies.
- Enjoining temple boards of trustees to get along with each other, to beware of detractors and to establish teaching programs for the youth.

RELIGIOUS STATESMANSHIP

- Providing a fearless, outspoken Hindu voice at interfaith conferences and spiritual and political forums, objecting to Christian hegemony at such gatherings, calling for equal representation by other religions, including the indigenous peoples, and decrying the hypocrisy of scientists who would speak as potential saviors for Earth's problems when science itself had caused many of the predicaments.
- Defending *advaitic* Śaiva Siddhānta at international conferences and with pundits of South Indian *aadheenams* to successfully affirm the legitimacy and antiquity of the nondual theology which so perfectly reflected his own realizations.
- Creating a method of ethical self-conversion for seekers to formally enter the Hindu religion, insisting that Hinduism has always accepted newcomers, refuting the notion that "You must be born a Hindu to be a Hindu."
- Encouraging people to practice their religion, whatever it may be, rather than nonreligious paths such as materialism, communism, existentialism and secular humanism.

PIONEERING PATTERNS

- Harnessing information technology to drive Hindu Dharma into the new millennium, including setting up the first Macintosh publishing network (1986) and founding the first major Hindu website (1994). In 1997 he launched TAKA, "Today at Kauai Aadheenam," to chronicle daily activities at his Kauai and Mauritius centers. He observed, "Now we have computers and the Internet—modern technology capable of bringing the spiritual beings and all religious people of the world closely together wherever they live. This one thing the typewriter could not do, the pen and paper could not do, the stylus and *olai* leaf did not do."

- Calling for the establishment of schools, *pāṭhaśālas*, to train temple priests outside of India.
- Promoting the idea of resident facilities for the elderly to live together close to temples in the West.
- Gifting Deity icons, usually of Gaṇeśa, to initiate the worship and remove obstacles at 36 temples globally.
- Establishing perpetual funds to finance his own and others' religious endeavors through Hindu Heritage Endowment.
- Finding ways for Hindus to meet cultural dilemmas in the modern age, such as devising a new festival, Pañcha Gaṇapati, celebrated for five days around the time of Christmas.
- Supporting cross-national marriages within his congregation and to the wider Hindu world.
- Drawing from the American church system to make his organization, and other Hindu institutions, socially viable, legally strong and structurally effective.
- Encouraging selfless, religious giving of one's time, resources and finances, and establishing tithing as a monthly practice within his global congregation.
- Establishing Innersearch Travel Study as a means of self-discovery and spiritual renewal for devotees and students, with his last three journeys consecrating new temples in Alaska, Trinidad and Denmark.
- Distinguishing outstanding leadership with his Hindu of the Year award.
- Introducing to Kauai: Toggenberg goats, Jersey cows, the honey bee industry and many species of exotic flora.

REVIVING NOBLE TRADITIONS

- Bringing sacraments, *saṁskāras*, back into vogue through his writings and by implementing them among his congregation with reverence and formal documentation.
- Campaigning for priests' rights and fair treatment, demanding they receive the same respect enjoyed by the clergy of other religions.
- Supporting and reviving the traditional arts, especially South Indian painting, with which he illustrated his trilogy; Indian dance, which he and his followers learned and taught; temple architecture, which he embodied in Iraivan Temple; Vedic astrology, which he used daily for its insights into character of people and timing of events; and *āyurveda,* which he promoted in his publications and encouraged as a natural healing system for his followers.
- Rescuing the home shrine from extinction—"out of the closet, into the most beautiful room of the home."

STRENGTHENING MONASTICISM

- Garnering respect for Hindu monastics of every order when "*swāmī* bashing" was common, proclaiming that *swāmīs* and *sādhus* are the ministers of this noble faith and that genuine *gurus* should be venerated, obeyed and sought out for their wisdom.
- Creating a global enclave of several hundred Hindu leaders and regularly calling on them for their wisdom on critical issues, from abortion, to cloning, to medical ethics and Hindu family life, publishing their collective views in HINDUISM TODAY.
- Breathing new life into the *aadheenams* of South India (temple-monastery complexes), bringing new

prominence to the Saṅkarāchārya centers and to the seats of power of all monastic lineages.
- Codifying in his *Holy Orders of Sannyāsa* the ideals, vows and aspirations of Hindu monasticism in unprecedented clarity and detail.

IMPROVING FAMILY LIFE

- Upholding the integrity of the family, extolling the extended family, finding ways to keep families close and harmonious, declaring that divorce is never a happy solution to marital conflict.
- Denouncing and taking action against wife abuse as a despicable act that no man has the right to perpetrate.
- Insisting on "zero tolerance for disharmonious conditions" within his monasteries and the homes of followers.
- Protecting children from abuse, standing up for their right to not be beaten by parents or teachers and debunking the notion that corporal punishment is a part of Hindu culture.
- Helping parents raise children with love and respect through Positive Discipline classes taught by his family devotees as a primary service to the community.
- Establishing a counter "women's liberation movement," reminding Hindus that family well-being lies in the hands of women, who with their special *śakti* are uniquely able raise their children well and make their husbands successful by not working in the world, but following the traditional role of wife and mother.

SETTING STANDARDS IN LEADERSHIP

- Creating Kauai Aadheenam, a temple-monastery in Hawaii so traditional and spiritual—replete with two Śiva temples, a large monastic order and a *satguru pīṭha* (seat of authority), all amid religious art, sculpture, traditional temple architecture and liturgy—that it stands as the most authoritative *aadheenam* in the West.
- Manifesting Iraivan, the first all-stone Āgamic temple in the West.
- Initiating and nurturing a traditional order of two dozen celibate Śaiva monastics, molding them into an effective, harmonious, traditional multi-national team.
- Building two platforms: Hindu solidarity, which he promoted through HINDUISM TODAY, and monistic Śaiva Siddhānta, which he elucidated in his eloquent and prolific publications.
- Being always available: personally greeting thousands of Hindu visitors to his *aadheenam*, speaking with them about their lives, concerns and aspirations.
- Fulfilling the motto "Think globally, act locally," joining monthly with Kauai leaders in an island visioning group to help manifest an enhanced social and economic future.

There are a few unusual men who have had enough of worldliness and choose to dance, live and merge with Śiva as Hindu monks.

These rare souls follow the path of the traditional Hindu monastic, vowed to poverty, humility, obedience, purity and confidence. They pursue the disciplines of *charyā, kriyā, yoga* and *jñāna* that lead to Self Realization. Knowing God is their only goal in life, the power that drives them tirelessly on. They live with other *maṭhavāsis* like themselves in monasteries, apart from worldliness, to worship, meditate, serve and realize the truths of the *Vedas* and *Śaiva Āgamas.* Guided by Satguru Bodhinatha Veylanswami, successor to Satguru Sivaya Subramuniyaswami, and headquartered at Kauai Aadheenam in Hawaii, USA, on the beautiful Garden Island of Kauai, the Saiva Siddhanta Yoga Order is among the world's foremost traditional Śaivite Hindu monastic orders, accepting candidates from every nation on Earth. It is an advaitic Śaiva Siddhānta order, a living stream of the ancient Nandinātha Sampradāya, originally deriving from India, and in recent centuries based in Sri Lanka. Young men considering the renunciate path who strongly believe they have found their spiritual calling in this lineage are encouraged to write to Bodhinatha, sharing their personal history, spiritual aspirations, thoughts and experiences. Holy orders of *sannyāsa* may be conferred on those who qualify after ten to twelve years of training. Write to:

Satguru Bodhinatha Veylanswami
Guru Mahāsannidhānam, Kauai Aadheenam
107 Kaholalele Road, Kapaa, Hawaii 96746-9304 USA
E-mail: Bodhi@hindu.org
World Wide Web: www.Gurudeva.org

The Hindu Heritage Endowment

Hindu thought and culture thread through almost every civilization on the planet, weaving a subtle tapestry of lofty philosophy and earthy, pragmatic wisdom. Whose life has not been touched? Some have been raised in India and enjoy memories of warm extended families and cool temples resounding with ancient *mantras*. Others find peace of mind in Hindu *yoga* practices. Many find solace in the concepts of *karma, dharma* and reincarnation, which express their own inner findings and beliefs. If you are one who has been touched by Hindu thought and culture, you may wish to further enrich your life by giving back to Sanātana Dharma in countries around the globe and helping preserve its rich heritage for future generations. ¶Hindu Heritage Endowment (HHE) provides such an opportunity. A public charitable trust recognized by the United States government, HHE was created to maintain permanent endowments for Hindu projects and institutions worldwide. Its endowments benefit orphanages, children's schools, *āśramas* and temples. They support priests and publish books; and they are designed to continue giving that financial support year after year, decade after decade, century after century. Whether you are inspired to give a few dollars to support orphanages or bequest millions in your will, write, give us a call or look us up on the Internet. Find out how to enrich your life by helping to preserve the treasures of a profound heritage for generations now living or as yet unborn.

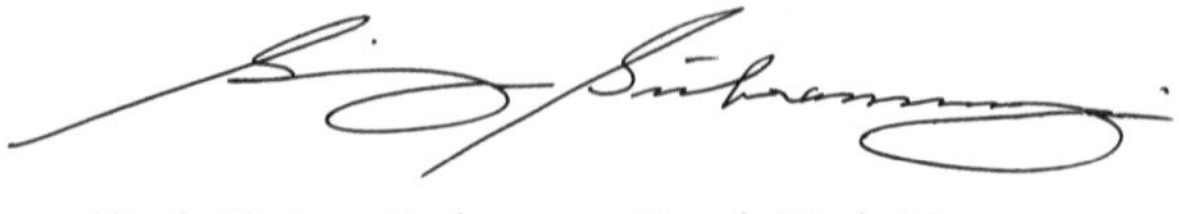

Hindu Heritage Endowment, Kauai's Hindu Monastery
107 Kaholalele Road, Kapaa, Hawaii, 96746-9304, USA.
Phone: (800) 890-1008; Outside of the US: (808) 822-3012, ext. 228
Fax: (808) 822-3152; E-mail: HHE@hindu.org
World Wide Web: www.HHEonline.org

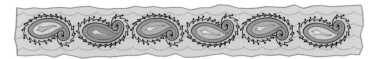

The Mini-Mela Giftshop

For all our books, visit store.himalayanacademy.com

Dancing with Śiva

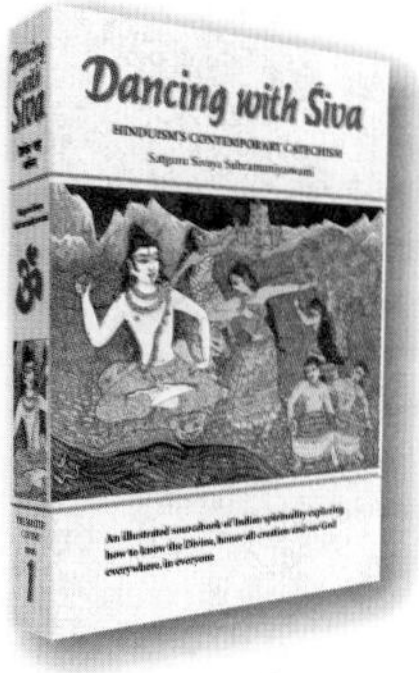

Hinduism's Contemporary Catechism
Book 1 of The Master Course Trilogy
By Satguru Sivaya Subramuniyaswami

This remarkable 1,000-page sourcebook covers every subject, answers every question and quenches the thirst of the soul for knowledge of God and the Self. Clearly written and lavishly illustrated, expertly woven with 600 verses from the *Vedas, Āgamas* and other holy texts, 165 South Indian paintings, 40 original graphics, a 25-page timeline of India's history and a 100-plus-page lexicon of English, Sanskrit and Tamil. A spiritual gem and great value at twice the price. "The most comprehensive and sensitive introduction to the living spiritual tradition of Hinduism, ...a feast for the heart and the mind (Georg Feuerstein)." Sixth edition, 2003, 7" x 10", full color, case bound (ISBN 0-945497-96-2), US$59.95.

Living with Śiva

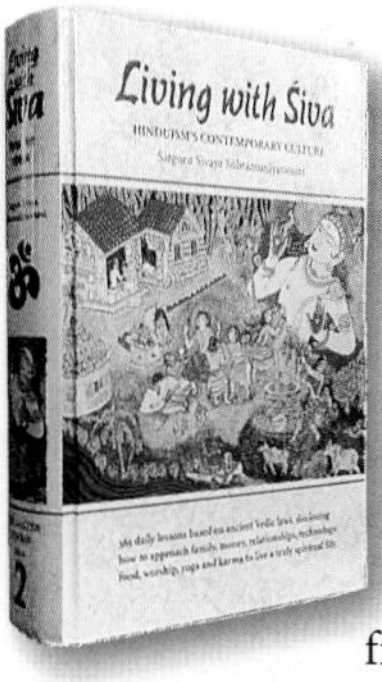

Hinduism's Contemporary Culture
Book 2 of The Master Course Trilogy
By Satguru Sivaya Subramuniyaswami

In the same bold, candid style of *Merging with Śiva,* Gurudeva focuses here on Hinduism's twenty restraints and observances that when dynamically applied bring order in life and establish a foundation for spirituality, meditation and realization. He addresses frankly and offers sound advice on the various problematic areas of modern living. The book is conveniently structured in 365 daily lessons disclosing how to approach family, money, relationships, technology, food, worship, *yoga* and *karma* to live a truly spiritual life. Second edition, beautiful full color art throughout, *haṭha yoga* and religious dues resources. Second edition, 2001, 7" x 10", case bound (ISBN 0-945497-98-9), US$59.95.

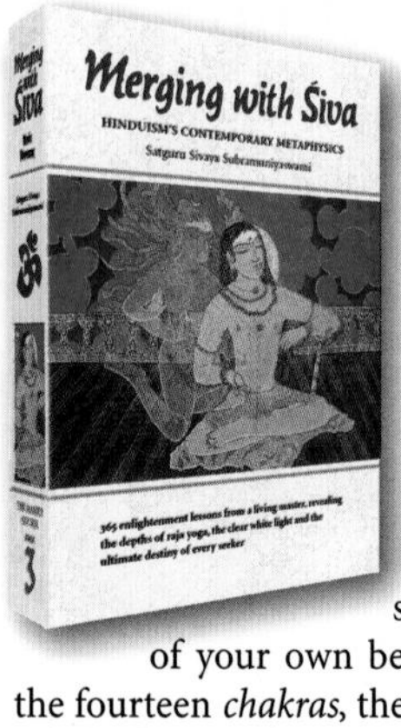

Merging with Śiva

Hinduism's Contemporary Metaphysics
Book 3 of The Master Course Trilogy
By Satguru Sivaya Subramuniyaswami

Here is the ultimate text for the really serious seeker. It may well go down in history as the richest and most inspired statement of meditation and God Realization ever, in any language. Yet, it's user-friendly, easy to follow, sensible and nonacademic! *Merging with Śiva* is 365 daily lessons, one for each day of the year, about the core of your own being. It's about God, about the mystical realm of the fourteen *chakras*, the human aura, *karma,* force fields, thought and the states of mind, the two paths, *samādhi* and so much more. Illustrated with fifty original South Indian paintings. Second edition, 2001, 1,000 pages, 7" x 10", case bound (ISBN 0-945497-99-7), US$59.95.

Loving Gaṇeśa

Hinduism's Endearing Elephant-Faced God
By Satguru Sivaya Subramuniyaswami

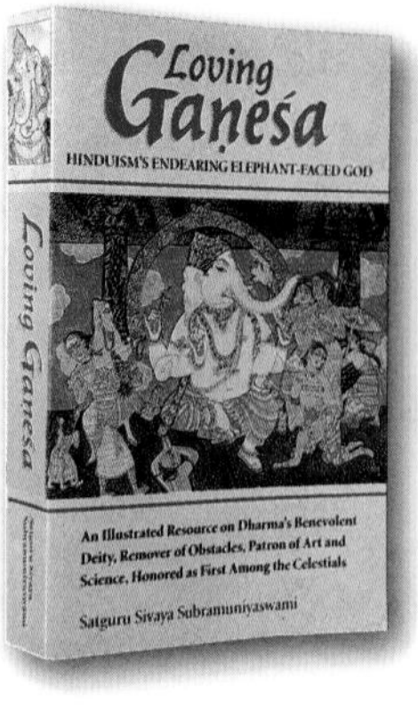

No book about this beloved elephant-faced God is more soul-touching. The Lord of Dharma will come to life for you in this inspired masterpiece. It makes approaching this benevolent Lord easy and inspiring. Learn about Gaṇeśa's powers, pastimes, *mantras,* nature, science, forms, sacred symbols, milk-drinking miracle and more. "A copy of *Loving Gaṇeśa* should be placed in every library and Hindu home"(Sri Om Prakash Sharma). Second edition, 1999, 576 pages, 5½" 8½", softcover (ISBN 0-945497-77-6), US$29.85.

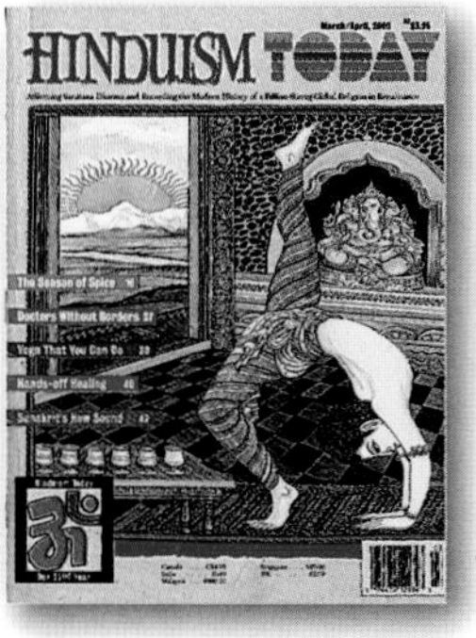

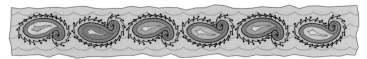

Hinduism Today

The International Magazine

Enjoy a spiritual experience with the foremost international journal on Sanātana Dharma, published by Satguru Bodhinatha Veylanswami and the *swāmīs* of the Saiva Siddhanta Yoga Order. Breaking news, ancient wisdom, modern trends, world-class photos, family resources, humor—you'll treasure every issue! "Hinduism Today is a beautiful example of the positive possibility of the media being fulfilled, a bright ray of light in a darkened world" (Anne Shannon, Portland). Introductory offer (US only): one-year subscription, four stunning issues, for US$35! And yes, the author of this book founded this global magazine and guided it for 20 years. ISSN 0896-0801; UPC: 0-74470-12134-3. Visit: www.HinduismToday.com

How to Become a Hindu

A Guide for Seekers and Born Hindus
By Satguru Sivaya Subramuniyaswami

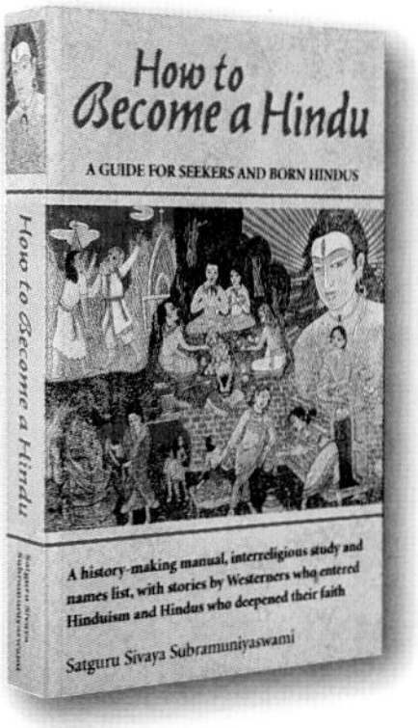

Hundreds of thousands of half-Hindus, having received a first name of a God or Goddess from their *yoga* teacher or a *swāmī*, want to enter the religion fully. Because of Hinduism's liberal doctrine, it is left to the individual as a "do-it-yourself conversion." How to Become a Hindu explains how the six steps of ethical conversion have enhanced the lives of many in the East and West. Here Americans, Canadians and Europeans tell their stories of passage from Western faiths to Hinduism. The book raises and convincingly settles the debate about non-Hindus entering the religion. "This elucidative book will provide immense help to those who wish to enter the Hindu fold, and also the younger generation of Hindus living outside India" (Puri Shankaracharya). First edition, 2000, 496 pages, 8½" x 5½", softcover (ISBN 0-945497-82-2), US$27.95.

Lemurian Scrolls

Angelic Prophecies Revealing Human Origins
By Satguru Sivaya Subramuniyaswami

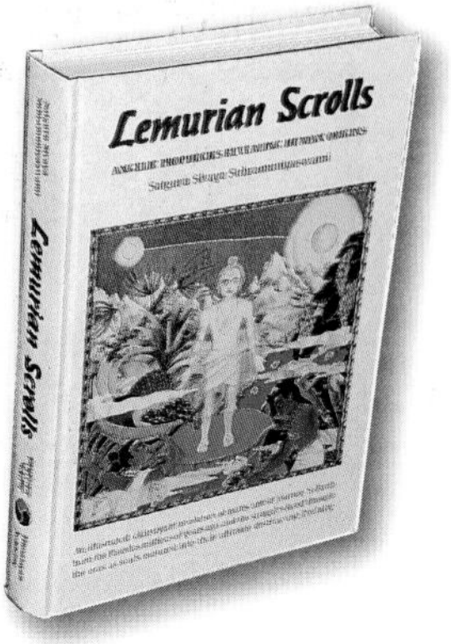

Enliven your spiritual quest with this clairvoyant revelation of mankind's journey to Earth millions of years ago from the Pleiades and other planets to further the soul's unfoldment. Learn about the ensuing challenges and experiences faced in evolving from spiritual bodies of light into human form and the profound practices followed and awakenings achieved in ancient Lemuria. These angelic prophecies, read by Sivaya Subramuniyaswami from *ākāśic* records written two million years ago, will overwhelm you with a sense of your divine origin, purpose and destiny and motivate a profound rededication to your spiritual quest. An extraordinary metaphysical book which answers the great questions: Who am I? Where did I come from? Where am I going? First Edition, 1998, 7½" x 10½", 400 pages, beautifully illustrated with original drawings, smythe-sewn and case bound with printed color cover (ISBN 0-945497-70-9), US$29.85.

Dancing with Śiva Pocketbook

Hinduism's Contemporary Catechism
NEW POCKETBOOK EDITION!
By Satguru Sivaya Subramuniyaswami

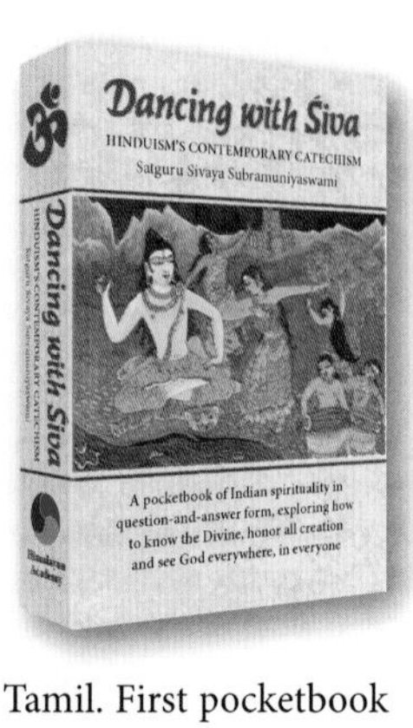

Now, carry the fullness of Hindu Dharma in your shirt pocket or purse. This remarkable little gem brings forward the same 155 questions and answers on contemporary Hindu philosophy, culture and metaphysics that have become world-renowned for the clear, practical way in which they explain the world's oldest religion to the modern seeker. Interwoven with verses from the *Vedas, Āgamas* and other holy texts, over 60 original graphics, a summary of Śaivite Hindu beliefs and a 750-plus-term glossary of English, Sanskrit and Tamil. First pocketbook edition, 2003, 3" x 4½", paperback (ISBN 0-945497-89-x), US$4.95.

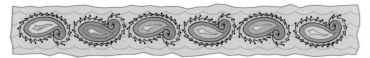

Order Form

☐ Please send me free literature.
☐ Send me an application for The Master Course Correspondence Study.
I wish to subscribe to HINDUISM TODAY. USA rates:
☐ 1 year, $35 ☐ 2 years, $65 ☐ 3 years, $95 ☐ Lifetime, $1001
(For international rates send e-mail to: subscribe@hindu.org)

I would like to order:

☐ *Dancing with Śiva*, $59.95
☐ *Living with Śiva*, $59.95
☐ *Merging with Śiva*, $59.95
☐ *How to Become a Hindu*, $27.95
☐ *Vedic Experience*, $39.75
☐ *Lemurian Scrolls*, $29.85
☐ *Loving Gaṇeśa*, $29.85
☐ *Dancing with Śiva Pocketbook*, $4.95

Prices are in US currency. Add 20% for postage and handling. Foreign orders are shipped sea mail unless otherwise specified and postage is paid. For foreign air mail, add 50% of the merchandise total for postage.

☐ My payment (check) is enclosed.
Please charge to my... ☐ MasterCard ☐ Visa ☐ Amex
Card number: __________________ Expiration, month:____ year:_____
Total of purchase: _______ Name on card: [PRINT] ____________________
Signature: ____
Address: [PLEASE PRINT] ____
____
Phone: ____________ Fax: ____________ E-mail: ______________

ORDER ON THE WEB AT store.HimalayanAcademy.com

OR MAIL, PHONE, FAX OR E-MAIL ORDERS TO:
Himalayan Academy Publications, Kauai's Hindu Monastery, 107 Kaholalele Road, Kapaa, Hawaii 96746-9304 USA. Phone (USA and Canada only): 1-800-890-1008; outside USA: 1-808-822-7032, ext. 238; Fax: 1-808-822-3152; E-mail: books@hindu.org

ALSO AVAILABLE THROUGH (write or call for prices):

Sanatana Dharma Publications, 15 Lintang Besi, Off Jalan Melawis, 41000 Klang, Selangor, Malaysia. Phone: 603-3371-9242. E-mail: chudika@tm.net.my

Sanathana Dharma Publications, Block 210 #06-326, Pasir Ris Street 21, Singapore 510210. Phone: 65-9664-9001; E-mail: sanatana@mbox4.singnet.com.sg

Saiva Siddhanta Church of Mauritius, La Pointe, Rivière du Rempart, Mauritius, Indian Ocean. Phone: 230-412-7177

Iraivan Temple Carving Site, P.O. Box No. 4083, Vijayanagar Main, Bangalore, 560 040. Phone: 91-80-839-7118; Fax: 91-80-839-7119; E-mail: jiva@vsnl.com

www.Gurudeva.org

Place
Stamp
Here

Mail to:

Satguru Bodhinatha Veylanswami
Kauai's Hindu Monastery
107 Kaholalele Road
Kapaa, Hawaii 96746–9304 USA

www.Gurudeva.org

Place
Stamp
Here

Mail to:

Satguru Bodhinatha Veylanswami
Kauai's Hindu Monastery
107 Kaholalele Road
Kapaa, Hawaii 96746–9304 USA

Yes! I am Interested!

Please place my name on your mailing list of registered owners of *Yoga's Forgotten Foundation:* I would like to receive a booklist of related publications, as well as an invitation to attend bookstore presentations, seminars and other events.

Name (PLEASE PRINT) ______________________

Address ______________________

____

City ______________ State ______________

Postal code ______________ Country ______________

Phone ______________ Fax ______________

E-mail ______________________

I have been studying the teachings of Satguru Sivaya Subramuniyaswami since ______________

Please check the items that apply to you:

- ☐ seeking a Hindu satguru
- ☐ studying various paths
- ☐ interested in joining one of Himalayan Academy's Travel-Study Programs
- ☐ considering life as a Hindu monk
- ☐ interested in subscribing to Hinduism Today magazine
- ☐ please send me information on the supervised correspondence study of *The Master Course*

Yes! I am Interested!

Please place my name on your mailing list of registered owners of *Yoga's Forgotten Foundation:* I would like to receive a booklist of related publications, as well as an invitation to attend bookstore presentations, seminars and other events.

Name (PLEASE PRINT) ______________________

Address ______________________

____

City ______________ State ______________

Postal code ______________ Country ______________

Phone ______________ Fax ______________

E-mail ______________________

I have been studying the teachings of Satguru Sivaya Subramuniyaswami since ______________

Please check the items that apply to you:

- ☐ seeking a Hindu satguru
- ☐ studying various paths
- ☐ interested in joining one of Himalayan Academy's Travel-Study Programs
- ☐ considering life as a Hindu monk
- ☐ interested in subscribing to Hinduism Today magazine
- ☐ please send me information on the supervised correspondence study of *The Master Course*